Nutrition Map

I0424760

ISBN-10: 1450500102
LCCN: 2010900086

Acknowledgments:

To my husband Eric:
You are my love, my soulmate, and my best friend. Together we have created a wonderful life. Thank you for always believing in me, and supporting me no matter what.

To my children:
You are my proudest achievements. I value, treasure, and enjoy every moment I spend with you.

To my mother:
You have taught me the importance of learning from all of life's experiences and how to be a strong person. You have made me the woman I am proud to be today.

To my aunt Aleida:
You have taught me the meaning of resilience and how to be an eternal optimist. Your everlasting support means the world to me.

Table of Contents

My gratitude goes to the individuals who have worked on this book, whether objectively providing feedback, designing it, translating it, or proofreading it. I would be remiss if I didn't mention their names and background:

Jose Antonio Sanabria R, M.D.
Internal Medicine & Infectious Diseases Specialist
Universidad Central
Caracas, Venezuela
and
Infectious Diseases Fellow
Harvard Medical University
Boston, Massachusetts, USA

Gaston Alcocer
Associate Degree, Graphic Design
Artistic Center Villasmil de Leon
Caracas, Venezuela

Maria Gabriela Kaiser
Masters Degree in Translation
Universidad Internacional de las Americas
San Jose, Costa Rica

Lydia R. Silva
B.Sc. Biology
University of Puerto Rico, Mayaguez Campus
Mayaguez, Puerto Rico

Foreword

Nutrition Map represents not only a very current attempt to face the problem of obesity but also a very pleasant conversation with a friend who sits in our home to tell us why it is worth changing our lifestyle, without suffering or feeling like victims.

Yvonne Quiñones Syto, our "new best friend," visits us with a simplicity that characterizes her and reaches deep into our souls! She bravely tells of her battle against weight gain and thus opens an interaction with us, the readers, who now finally have a real person who truly identifies with us.

Yvonne changes the paradigms of everything we hate about diets by introducing a new system based on small steps that we can all take. She shares small and big tips that make sense in our lives and which we can start to put into practice after finishing each chapter.

Finally, someone understands that "we love chocolate" and tells us when and how we should enjoy it without feeling tortured or unhappy.

This is a wonderful book, and it represents a real, accessible, and friendly source on which we can build our new and final plan against obesity.

Each page provides not only a glimpse of reality but also a hand that guides us through a road we knew existed but which we did not dare to take before.

Obesity is undoubtedly the number one enemy of our society. It is not only a dangerous condition per se but also the cause of the most serious consequences, both metabolic (hyperlipemia and diabetes) and cardiovascular (atherosclerosis, hypertension).

This condition has turned into a silent epidemic that impacts all races, genders, and ages and has dangerously spread in our population.

The media bombards us with images of delicious food in large portions and dangerously invites us to a world of delight. Contradictorily, it presents a mixed message of anorexic models wearing tiny sizes and creating in our minds a stressful controversy: "It's great to eat without limits, but you also have to be slim."

Yvonne, our friend, understands that we will probably never be runway models and that each pound we lose is a moment of celebration in our lives; and there lies the difference between *Nutrition Map* and other books in the market. Understanding that each inch and each pound are rewards is not easy for someone who does not understand the mindset of overweight patients. That is why it is essential that our friend has really found this colloquial, simple, and deep way to communicate with us.

By changing our bad habits, even those we were unaware of, we are building a solid foundation for a healthy life in which maybe the greatest reward is to achieve self-control. By exercising self-control, we can improve our health in a world in which we will still have to deal with facing tempting food choices and passion for food.

Yvonne releases us from that "bony and troubled" image and turns us into a better version of ourselves, with our likes and weaknesses. More importantly, she helps us to achieve an educated mindset that helps us to accept only what is beneficial for us.

Yvonne's broad experience in the field of nutrition provides us with the necessary weapons in our struggle, mainly in our ability to accept ourselves and be happy with the results of our small daily battles.

I am sure the readers will truly enjoy this book. *Nutrition Map* is a source to have handy when we need support, when the scale displays a number greater than the one we want, or when our pants do not feel as loose as we would like. More importantly it will be a source of inspiration when we are not able to say no but can make healthy choices to say yes, and thus enjoy eating with no remorse because we have made the right choices and are happy in doing so.

Jose Antonio Sanabria R, M.D.
Internal Medicine & Infectious Diseases Specialist

Preface

As a child, I wasn't considered one of the smallest children in the class; however, I wasn't the largest either, though I was one of the shortest. Around the fifth grade, my weight started to climb. For as long as I can recall, I was overweight, especially after I hit puberty. The numbers on the scale never corresponded to the numbers on the charts in the pediatrician's office.

Although I was overweight, at home, we followed a healthy lifestyle. If the weather was agreeable (meaning no rain), then I was outside playing with a friend from across the street. All of our meals were prepared at home, and we hardly ate out. Candy, cookies, cakes—well, basically any form of sugar—were allowed only on special occasions, such as Halloween. We were allowed soda only on the weekends, and if by Monday we had forgotten, then we had to wait until the following weekend. When we went to the supermarket, we could only buy what was on the coupon, and wouldn't you know it, candy was never on the coupon! I don't even remember there being juice in the house, just water or milk to drink.

When we were allowed treats, we had to brush our teeth soon after, which probably explains why I didn't get a cavity until I went away to college. From the age of five through at least to twelve or thirteen, I was enrolled in dance classes a few days a week, and my mother made sure that I was active. I never sat in front of the television for more than a half an hour or so. Despite all this, I was overweight, yet my parents never ever made a negative comment.

Although my mother seemed strict, I never gave the way we lived a second thought. It was just the way things were. The summer before I started high school, I decided that I wanted to get into shape and lose some weight. I was reading one of my mother's magazines and read about exercises I could do at home. I taped exercise shows (yes, on a VCR) and worked out to them every day. When possible, I would walk to a friend's house instead of getting a ride (at least a mile each way). I managed to drop fifteen pounds before school started, and I never looked back.

While researching what I wanted to be when I grew up in my sophomore year, I came across becoming a dietitian. You mean, I could spend the next four years studying what I loved to read about already? I could get paid to talk about food all day? Sign me up. Here I am, many years later, a registered dietitian (yeah, that four years was really five plus after the internship) still getting paid to talk about food all day long. In those years I have seen "diet" trends come and go. I have friends, family, and clients try every fad "diet" on the market, yet the majority of them ends up gaining the weight back and then some. Weight loss books are plentiful, but many do not provide sound nutrition advice. Ask most registered dietitians and they will agree: the solution is not to "diet"; rather, practice healthy habits and live an active lifestyle including exercise, and the rest will fall into place. So I present to you how to do it.

Introduction (Yes, You Must Read This Before the First Chapter)

As a registered dietitian (RD), I have been extensively trained as to how I am "supposed" to eat. More importantly, I have been taught how to teach *you* how to eat. But like many health care professionals, I was my own worst patient and did not follow my own advice. That changed one day when I received the results from my yearly physical. At the ripe old age of twenty-eight, I had a cholesterol level of 280 mg/dl and a triglyceride level well over the normal limit. Not good, considering my family history of high cholesterol, high blood pressure, and diabetes. That was my wake-up call. I had just gotten married and gained back the fourteen pounds that I struggled for six months to lose, then gained fifteen more for padding, and stopped exercising. I decided that I wanted to live a healthy life and live to see my grandchildren have children (or something like that).

Food is everywhere! Try to go through your hometown without finding at least one of every fast food chain. Within a six-mile radius of my home, one fast food establishment has four locations. Quite a difficult task to avoid them, wouldn't you say? Try to find a holiday that isn't surrounded by food. When you go to a friend's house, food is usually the first thing offered to you. When you plan a get together what is the first thing you think of: *What will I serve?* Food is pleasurable and a social experience for human beings. It brings people together. It will always be everywhere, so it is time to live with it and enjoy it.

Food: consume it...don't let it consume you.

A few questions before I begin:

- Do you feel like you are constantly on a "diet"?

- Are you on a "diet" more than you are off of one?

- How many "diet plans" have you been on?

- How old were you when you started dieting?

- Have you tried all of the programs out there without any continued success?

- Are you wondering why none of these "diets" work for the long term?

According to a study conducted in 2004, obesity is the second cause of death in the United States, second only to tobacco, causing approximately 400,000 deaths in the year 2000.[1] In comparison, tobacco related deaths caused approximately 435,000 deaths.[1] What is even more alarming is that the number of adults succumbing to this preventable cause of death will increase by an estimated 15,000 deaths per year.[1] Obesity leads to diseases including diabetes, heart disease, elevated cholesterol and triglycerides, cancer, hypertension, gallstones, sleep apnea, osteoarthritis, and gynecological problems.[2]

Right along with the rising obesity rates, there is an abundance of weight loss "diets" and "diet" products out on the market that promise unbelievable results in record time. If you have tried any of these "diets," you may have noticed that many of them actually work; that is, if you are able to stay on them. Some even produce amazing results. Let's review several of the popular "diets" out there.

1. The cabbage soup diet: This "diet" is a classic. It boasts that "you'll lose weight fast" while eating as much as you want. The catch is that the eating as much as you want only applies to the foods on a list provided. Also, you can't be on the program for longer than seven days. So if you have a substantial amount of weight to lose, this is probably not the plan for you. However, the Web site points out that the "diet" can be utilized as a "kick-start for a more moderate diet." Hmmm, "moderate diet." What does that mean? Side effects include light-headedness, weakness, and decrease in concentration (sure sounds like a commercial for prescription medication, doesn't it?), but the Web site asserts that these side effects are well worth it because of the results—and you only have to suffer for seven days. Seven days of headaches, by choice? I think not.[3]

2. "High-protein diets," also known as "low-carb "diets": These diets come in many forms; however, their basic principle is that carbohydrates, or carbs for short, are bad for your waistline. Carbs are limited; however, some plans exclude them all together. While carbohydrates in these plans are considered the enemy, protein, fats, and some vegetables are your friends. So if you dislike foods like breads, cereal, rice, pasta, fruit, milk, or yogurt, this may be the plan for you. I am an old-fashioned Cuban girl married to a Chinese man. No beans and rice? Not happening in my house.

3. Fat-free "diet" craze: Sit back and think back to the early 1990s. Remember the fat-free craze? Low-fat and nonfat foods were all the rage. Most importantly, there

was fat-free ice cream. Now that you have taken out all of the fat, why is it that you still aren't losing any weight? What went wrong? Low-fat "diets" can work to help you lose weight. However, reducing fat isn't the only change that will make you lose weight. Many of the low- and nonfat foods on the market still have the same amount of calories as their regular counterparts. When you take the fat out of a recipe, you have to put something back in. Many products have added sugar or protein for texture and flavor, which adds calories. Remember, a calorie is a calorie. No matter where the source of the calorie (a carbohydrate, protein, or fat), when you eat more than your body needs in a day, you will gain weight. So if you now follow a low-fat meal plan, if you are still consuming more calories than your body needs, you will not lose weight; and you may even gain weight. More on that later.

4. The Replacements: Depending on the manufacturer of the product you intend to use, these "diets" basically require the replacement of two meals per day with meal replacement shakes or bars. Some plans only instruct you to consume shakes and bars for the first few weeks. I don't know about you, but the majority of the time, I enjoy chewing my meals and not just drinking them.

So if many of these "diets" claim to work, why are more and more people fighting the battle of the bulge? Despite the abundance of "diet" plans and weight loss products on the market, the fact is that people are just getting bigger. So what is the problem?

A fad "diet" is a short-lived way of eating that often has a cult following. Many start these trendy "diets" and follow them religiously. Often, these diets, like history, are doomed to repeat themselves throughout time. For example, when the low carb "diet" craze became all the rage again, I had just become a dietitian. I was working in a small community hospital dealing mostly with patients with cardiac problems. I had numerous patients flat out refuse to have toast with their morning eggs, or mashed potatoes with their baked chicken. Despite just suffering a heart attack or stroke, they still want extra butter.

Most of the time people lose weight quickly on these "diets," and that is why they become popular. People lose weight as long as they stick to them exactly as recommended. Much of the weight is lost quickly in the first few days or weeks.

The trouble with fad "diets" is that they are pretty difficult to stick to, usually because they are often unrealistic. Usually, the weight that is lost is gained back once the "diet" is discontinued. What makes it worse are the bonus pounds gained in addition to the original weight that was lost. The reason: because the "diets" have failed to educate people on how to live once off the "diet." So if you are just going to gain all the weight back once you have worked so hard to lose it, why bother following a "diet"?

If it sounds too good to be true, then it probably is too good to be true. If we could all have a perfect body in just three minutes a day, then there wouldn't be so many overweight people in this country. If you could keep off those ten pounds you lost in two days with the miraculous liquid "diets" available, there would be a lot fewer overweight people struggling to lose weight. If it only took one pill each day, everyone would be thinner, right?

Any plan that eliminates whole food groups or remotely suggests that it can change your genetic makeup is not going to work. There are no good or bad foods when it comes to weight loss. There is no one super food that will cause weight loss, and no one food that is the main culprit in weight gain. Read them for a good laugh and then move on. Be especially careful if they say that their "diet" is based on years of research. Often, the creators of these studies take one line from a large study and run with it without waiting for more studies to be done that repeat the results. Be especially cautious if the plan encourages the use of special products in conjunction with the plan. They are basically just trying to sell a product and could care less if it actually works or not. The goal is to make a buck or two.

You may have noticed that I use the word "diet" in quotes. In my lifetime, I have come to think of the word "diet" for what it is: a horrible four-letter word that should be banned. Just like the words we forbid children to use, the word "diet" should be eliminated from your vocabulary.

I am not suggesting that you follow a "diet" in the weight loss sense. What I want you to take away from this book is a new way of living and eating. I want you to wake up in the morning and not dread mealtimes. I want you to enjoy food. Lord knows I do. Heck, I became a dietitian because I love food. I have one of the best jobs in the world. Basically, I get paid to talk about food. After you are done reading this book, I want you to start living and stop struggling. You are about to begin relearning how to eat well and plan your meals. This plan is different. It isn't even a "diet."

Part I:
Learning the Basics

Motivation

If you have not read the introduction section, please go back and do so. If you have already completed the reading, please proceed.

- Want to fit into that bikini this summer?

- "Skinny" pants all the rage, and you just can't imagine getting into them with your hips and thighs?

- Getting together with old high school friends and want to make sure you're as thin as you were back then?

- Have a bet going with your buddies about who can lose the most weight?

- Want to get back into the jeans you wore before you were pregnant?

- Are you trying to make an impression at the next holiday party?

- Are you tired of feeling out of breath when you go up a flight of stairs?

- Do you want to be more active outdoors with the kids?

- Do you want to keep up with the grandkids?

- Would you like to try to lower your cholesterol without having to immediately depend on the use of medications?

- Do you want to try to get rid of the back pains that have progressively gotten worse and worse as the numbers on the scale have crept up?

What was your motivation to read this book? Was it for similar reasons to those listed above? Motivation is what drives you to initiate changes in your behavior. Motivation for changing your eating habits can be stirred by simply looking at an old picture of yourself or getting the results from a medical exam. Making changes in your eating plan is going to be a long-term investment.

Before you begin making changes:

1. Find a nice notebook or create a file in your PDA, laptop, or desktop computer and title it **"GOALS."**

2. Make a list of your reasons for losing weight. Really think about why you want to make changes.

3. Examine your reasons.

Are they realistic goals? If you are a size 18, setting your sites on being a size 2 is setting yourself up for a nose dive into a pint of ice cream. Now, planning to get down to a size 16 within three months' time...that's more like it. For example, some realistic goals would sound like:

- I will be able to exercise every other day for at least thirty minutes.

- I will have at least two fruits and two vegetables every day.

- I will try a new physical activity each month.

  o Month 1: Yoga

  o Month 2: Hiking

  o Month 3: Volleyball

- I will lower my cholesterol by ten points.

You get the picture. Think in the long term. Not just in the now.

Make sure you are making these changes for you and no one else. If you are trying to lose weight to have a "bikini body" this summer, then watch out, you're about to fall off the plan. If you are doing this to get someone to notice you, then this isn't really for you.

Stick to the plan and always remember what the ultimate goal is: to lead a healthier lifestyle and ward off health problems in the future. These are changes to last a lifetime. The truth is, when you set your goals on the short term, you set yourself up for a fall. Constantly reevaluate your incentives to make changes.

Getting Started

Disclaimer

- Before making any changes in your daily meal plan, please consult with your physician or health care provider for clearance.

- The information presented in this book is intended to help you make informed decisions about your meal plan and health. This material is not intended to be a substitute for medical counseling. Have a regular checkup to make sure that there aren't any medical conditions that you didn't know about.

- All of the information presented in this book is for educational purposes only. For individual recommendations, discuss a referral to a registered dietitian with your primary health care provider (and check out www.eatright.org to find a registered dietitian in your area).

- There are no forbidden foods in this meal plan; however, that does not mean that you can go to town and have fried foods all day long or a piece of pie after every meal.

In your weight loss file created earlier, create a new file or page and label it "STARTING STATISTICS." Bring this to your physician or health care provider and have them help you fill in some of the information below. This is especially helpful to keep as a record when you go to new physicians or other health care providers (see table 1).

Table 1: Starting Statistics   Date:_____

Table 1: Starting Statistics   Date:_____

Height: _____   Weight: _____   Goal Weight: _____

Blood Pressure: _____ Fasting Blood Sugar:_____

Total Cholesterol: _____

HDL Cholesterol: _____   LDL Cholesterol: _____

Other pertinent laboratory data:

_____

_____

Pertinent Medical History:

_____

_____

_____

Pertinent Surgical History:

_____

_____

_____

Current Medications:

_____

_____

_____

Vitamins:	Supplements:
_____	_____
_____	_____
_____	_____

Do not expect to lose an obscene amount of weight quickly. Basically, if you have thirty pounds to lose, don't expect that this plan with melt it away in a matter of six weeks. Weight lost too quickly will likely be regained even faster than it was lost, usually with some bonus pounds.

How the Plan Works

So this is how the plan is going to work. This book is set up as a series of chapters which are designed for you to follow at your own pace. Ideally you want to work through each chapter in about one week's time. However, if you find that you have been able to make the suggested changes faster than the suggested week and would like to proceed to the next chapter before the week is out, then go for it. When possible, though, try to take the whole week to make the changes. Don't go through the tasks too quickly.

Weight loss, true weight loss, and weight maintenance take time. The longer it takes you to take the weight off, the longer you will keep it off. We want long-lasting results. What is the cliché? Rome wasn't built in a day. The same holds true here. All of the weight won't come off in a day.

Just as you'll be able to breeze through some of the chapters in this book, some chapters may take longer than a week. If that happens, then so be it. Some tasks are a bit more challenging than others. Each and every person is different. Each person has different cravings, food aversions, and weaknesses. For example, it may be easier for you to have more fruit than vegetables. The vegetable chapter may take you some time, and that is OK; just make sure that you make the changes. Do this at your own pace, but do complete the task. Try not to get stuck for weeks at a time. Do move on and conquer more tasks. It is all up to you.

The plan also works in another way. As you proceed to each tip, you build on what you have learned. For example, first you learned your alphabet way back in the day. Next, you learned how to read small words like *cat* and *dog*. Then the words became bigger and bigger until you could read a whole book. As you went on in the process, you always remembered the alphabet you first learned and built on the lessons from there.

This works in precisely the same way. If one week you are to eat two or more fruits each day and the following week I recommend two vegetables per day, that doesn't mean that you no longer have to eat fruit. Yup, now you must eat two or more fruits and two or more vegetables each and every day...you'll see.

Week 1 Beginners' Tips

Your first week on the plan seems simple enough: exercise a couple of days each week, drink plenty of water, and keep a log of it all. These three tips are to set you up to follow the most valuable advice that anyone can give you about living healthy. The trick is not just knowing what the three tips are but actually following them, forever! That is right, my friend, I said forever.

Tip 1: Keeping a Journal

Start keeping a journal, a food journal, that is. The best way to make progress is by keeping track of what changes you are making and periodically reviewing the journal as you go. Keeping a log of what you're eating will ultimately help you become more aware of your eating habits, and help you pinpoint where you can make changes for a healthier lifestyle.

Start by finding a food journal that fits your lifestyle. Ideally, choose something that is pocket sized so that you can carry it around with you, and so you won't forget to write things down later.

You can use:

- A small notebook.

- Index cards that you carry throughout the day and put in a recipe box at the end of the day.

- An pocket organizer (paper or electronic).

39

Whatever you choose is fine as long as you keep the food journal up to date each and every day.

<u>What to record</u> (see table 2):
- The time you ate.

- What you ate.

- How much you ate.

<u>You can also include:</u>

- Approximately how long it took you to eat.

- Any significant feelings associated with eating that meal, snack, or food item.

- Exercise done (type of activity and duration).

- Grocery shopping lists.

- Monthly weight.
  - *This should be done only once a month (at the most) at the same time each month (i.e., the first of every month).*

- Measurements (see table 3).
  - *This should be done only once a month (at the most) at the same time each week (i.e., every Monday).*

Do not weigh yourself every day. Your weight can fluctuate from day to day. If you weighed 183 pounds yesterday and weigh 184 today, it could set you up for a downfall if you are sensitive to the numbers. NOTE: If weighing yourself every week bothers you, then don't do it! Maybe taking your measurements is a better idea and may be more indicative than the scale of how you are doing on your exercise and meal plan. If taking your measurements as well, do so once a month (see table 3). For anyone with a history of an eating disorder(s), I strongly recommend that you avoid the scale. Stick with writing in a journal only.

Table 2: Journal   Date:_____

Breakfast	Time:_____	Snack 1	Time:_____
_____		_____	
_____		_____	
_____		_____	
_____		_____	

Lunch	Time:_____	Snack 2	Time:_____
_____		_____	
_____		_____	
_____		_____	
_____		_____	

Dinner	Time:_____	Snack 3	Time:_____
_____		_____	
_____		_____	
_____		_____	
_____		_____	

Exercise:	Water Consumed:
_____	☐☐☐☐ ☐☐☐☐ ☐☐☐☐
_____	Other Beverages:
_____	_____
_____	_____

Shopping List:	Comments:
_____	_____
_____	_____
_____	_____
_____	_____

Table 3: Measurements

Table 3: Measurements

Starting Date: _____

Height: _____   Starting Weight: _____

Date:_____ Bicep:_____ Bust:_____ Waist:_____ Hips:_____ Thigh:_____ Calf _____	Date:_____ Bicep:_____ Bust:_____ Waist:_____ Hips:_____ Thigh:_____ Calf _____	Date:_____ Bicep:_____ Bust:_____ Waist:_____ Hips:_____ Thigh:_____ Calf _____
Date:_____ Bicep:_____ Bust:_____ Waist:_____ Hips:_____ Thigh:_____ Calf _____	Date:_____ Bicep:_____ Bust:_____ Waist:_____ Hips:_____ Thigh:_____ Calf _____	Date:_____ Bicep:_____ Bust:_____ Waist:_____ Hips:_____ Thigh:_____ Calf _____
Date:_____ Bicep:_____ Bust:_____ Waist:_____ Hips:_____ Thigh:_____ Calf _____	Date:_____ Bicep:_____ Bust:_____ Waist:_____ Hips:_____ Thigh:_____ Calf _____	Date:_____ Bicep:_____ Bust:_____ Waist:_____ Hips:_____ Thigh:_____ Calf _____

Comments:_____

_____

_____

Tip 2: Water

Drink eight to twelve cups of water each day, especially if you are starting an exercise program unless otherwise directed by your health care provider.

Water has many functions including:

- Keeps your body functioning properly and smoothly.

- Helps to eliminate wastes and toxins in the body.

- Helps to maintain soft skin.

- Keeps electrolytes in check.

- Can help keep you feeling full.

- Helps to regulate temperature body whether you live in hot or cold climates.

- Cushions and protects your joints.

- And don't forget, it is calorie, fat, cholesterol, caffeine and sodium free.

Getting started:

- Don't wait until you are thirsty. Usually by this point it is too late, so drink water all of the time!

- Carry a one-liter bottle of water every day and drink two each day, or carry a sixteen-ounce bottle of water every day and drink four each day.

- Drink seltzer flavored with lemon or lime.

- Drink before, during, and after exercising.

- Drink one full glass before meals to increase fullness so you don't overeat.

- Non-caffeinated beverages do count (caffeinated and alcoholic beverages don't count because they may dehydrate you).

Tip 3: Exercise

Exercise for thirty minutes at a time, three to five days each week (yes, each and every week). Eventually you want to work up to exercising four to five days a week allowing for breaks throughout the week. The United States Department of Agriculture actually reports that sixty to ninety minutes of daily physical activity may be needed to prevent weight gain and maintain weight loss.[4] Pick a time that you know you will do it. If you know you need to exercise right after waking up so you won't put it off, then that is the time you should do it. You get the idea. Just make sure it's OK with your doctor before you start. Remember, exercise is just one of the steps to making healthy lifestyle changes, and by no means the only step.

Why Exercise?

- Helps preserve the muscle you have and help you build more while you're making healthy changes.

- *Preserving the muscle you already have will also help you maintain weight loss. "Muscle Management" is important so you don't regain the weight you worked so hard to lose. The more muscle you have, the more efficient your body is at burning calories. Thus, the more efficient your body is at losing weight.*

- Decreases the amount of fat mass in the body.

- Helps to protect your bones.

- Increases your immune function.

- Lowers the risks of diseases such as diabetes.

- May allow you to eat more.

- May help you sleep more easily so you need less sleep and feel refreshed when you wake up.

Getting started:

- To start, write down all of the reasons why you put off exercising in your journal (journal instructions to follow) and list ways to overcome these excuses.

- Keep a set of exercise clothes in the car at all times.

- Find activities that you enjoy doing.

- Find new forms of exercising to vary your routine so you don't get jaded. Join a yoga class. Go on hiking adventures.

- Park the car as far as possible from the door at the supermarket or mall.

- Walk! Drive only when you must.

- Put the video games down and get outside! It's a beautiful day (even if it is raining or freezing)!

- Instead of hiring a gardener, rake the leaves yourself.

- Take the stairs.

- When on vacation, look for hotels that have fitness centers or gyms and offer healthy meals. Even better, go on vacations to destinations where good health is the main objective.

Week 1 may take longer than one week, and that's fine. Try not to take too long. The best is yet to come. Write down everything you are eating and drinking, and log your workouts in your journal. At the end of the day, look back at what you have consumed. Don't beat yourself up if you overindulged at any point throughout the day. Check off any places where you find weaknesses and areas you can improve.

Week 2 Portion Sizes: Sometimes It Isn't What You Eat, But How Much

"I eat all of the 'right' foods, I just eat too many of them."

I may be a dietitian with many years of training, but I am human. I became a dietitian for the same reasons a chef becomes a chef: I love food! I love talking about it, preparing it, and of course, eating it. There aren't many foods I won't eat, and there aren't many foods I haven't at least tried. Like Mom always used to say, "How do you know you don't like it if you haven't tried it?" so I will always give new foods a chance.

Over the years, I have found that in order to enjoy some of my favorite foods I had to figure out a way to incorporate them into my daily meal plan without gaining weight each and every time I partake in an indulgence of "sometimes" foods.

Just like many of you reading this book, I wasn't blessed with a super-charged metabolism or even a slender build. I have to eat healthy and exercise. I don't lose weight quickly, but I can sure gain it quickly if I'm not careful. Like I said earlier, I love food. All food: the good, the bad, the ugly, and the delicious. Often when I talk to clients I find that they enjoy many of the so-called "right" foods. Perfect "diets" you think? Probably not the case. I have yet to have a client who follows a perfect "diet." Come to think of it, not many dietitians follow a perfect "diet," because there is no such thing.

So what's the problem? Remember, too much of a good thing isn't always good. Eating too much of a good thing can be a really bad thing. Weight gain basically comes from eating more calories than your body needs and expending less due to low physical activity.

Portions in the United States have increased dramatically over the past few years. Remember back in the good old days when the small serving of French fries in your favorite fast food restaurant was really a small size? They came in a small paper sleeve that is now located in the French fries of the children's meal. The adult small has become what we used to call the large size. Have times changed! If you are served one serving of juice, you may consider it a "shot" glass instead of a serving. In many locations it has become cheaper and cheaper to order the larger sizes, making it all too easy to go overboard. Why get a twelve-ounce soda when the thirty-ounce is only ten cents more?

So how can eating too many fruits or vegetables in a day be a bad thing? This is where a little thing called your metabolism comes into play. Simply put, your metabolism is the rate at which your body uses up energy. The rate at which a body uses up energy varies from one person to the next. Also, metabolism can change throughout a person's lifetime. For example, you burn energy at a much higher rate in your teens than in your forties. This explains why eating the same way you did in high school will slowly make the pounds creep on throughout the years.

The rate at which you burn energy can also be affected by your total calorie intake. Case in point: If your body needs 1800 calories a day to maintain your current weight and all of a sudden you start to consume 1000 calories a day, you will lose weight because you are eating less than your body needs for weight maintenance. However, over time the body will adjust and become accustomed to functioning on fewer calories, and the weight loss will cease. This is also known as a weight plateau. The unfortunate thing is, the day you have more than the 1000 calories, let's say 200 extra calories for 1200 total calories, you will start to gain weight. Your metabolism has dropped, and your body in essence is functioning more efficiently.

A calorie is a calorie no matter where it comes from. Calories do add up. If your body needs 1800 calories a day and you consistently have less than that, you will lose weight; have more than the 1800 calories, and you will gain weight. It doesn't matter where those calories come from. Excess calories get stored as fat. Lovely, isn't it? In order to lose a pound, you have to have a 3500-calorie deficit. Thus, if you reduce your calories by 250 each day, whether by eating less or by exercising, you will lose half a pound in a week. Cut back by five hundred calories each day, and you will lose about one pound per week.

Remember back to when we talked about fad "diets"? Many fad "diets" work because they eliminate one or more food groups. For example, low carbohydrate "diets" work mainly because three major food groups are being eliminated (starches, fruits, and milk/yogurt). When three groups are eliminated, many lose weight because they are consuming fewer calories. However, in my practice I have seen some lose the weight, and then gain it back when they start to bring back the carbs. Some even gain weight or remain the same, mainly because they have replaced the calories that came from carbohydrates with "allowed" foods.

With all this talk about calories, you may be thinking, "Does she expect me to start calculating how many calories I eat in a day?" Not exactly. Take a look back at your logbook. If you haven't been writing the amount of each food consumed, now is the time to start. If you have been writing the amounts consumed but have not been actually measuring, now is definitely the time to start.

Some guidelines to better portion control:

Invest in:

- A small kitchen scale to weigh foods. This is one of the most important tools that you can have in your kitchen. The scale is the best tool for learning what a real portion is. You will be amazed. There are two basic types for home use: digital and mechanical dials. Prices can range from $9.99-$99.99. I recommend that you invest in a digital display since they tend to be more user friendly and can measure in small increments.

- Next to the food scale, measuring cups are the most important tool that you need in your kitchen. Purchase a set of dry measuring cups to measure dry foods such as cereal and pasta, and a set of wet measuring cups to measure liquids like juices and soups. Wet measuring cups usually come in one-, two-, and four-cup increments. You can usually find sets of three for under twenty dollars. Truthfully, all you need is one in your kitchen that measures one cup at a time. Dry measuring cups usually come in sets and are made of stainless steal or plastic. Either will do.

- Measuring spoons are needed to measure fats and condiments (i.e. peanut butter, oils, and salad dressings). Usually, measuring spoons come in five-piece sets and can be purchased combined with dry measuring cups. Measuring spoons come in stainless steel or plastic. Some companies also have adjustable measuring spoons that measure one teaspoon up through one tablespoon. Either will do; however, the adjustable spoon is a good item for your lunch bag or purse for when you eat out. Prices depend on the material you use and can range from as little as $2.99 (or less) and up.

- Pocket nutrition guide. You could purchase this online; however, I highly recommend that you trek over to a local bookstore and review what is available. Usually they are located in the Health and Fitness section of the store. Try to choose one that is not persuading you to follow a specific "diet" plan. Instead, look for a guide that lists the serving size of a food with total calories, fat, total carbohydrates (with total fiber amount), and protein.

Reading a Food Label

The majority of foods in the United States are required to have a label that provides nutrition information. Use the label to learn what the correct portion sizes are for everything you eat, especially the foods you know you go overboard on. Head over to your kitchen cabinet or pantry and choose your favorite snack food.

For now you will focus on:

- The Serving Size: The serving size listed is for one serving. The measurement provided is in a typical household measurement (i.e., cups or number of pieces) and is followed by the metric weight for one serving. This is where the food scale will help. It is easier to measure one ounce of cheese crackers than counting out forty-five pieces of them.[5]

- The Servings per Container: Underneath the serving size is the amount of total servings in the package or container. Make sure to pay close attention to this on a label because many of the products you enjoy as one serving really have two or more servings.[5]

- Calories: This is the amount of calories in one serving, not in the total package or container.[5]

Tips:

- Weigh or measure portions until you are able to "eyeball" them. I have been a dietitian for over eight years and still measure many foods that I know I will go overboard on. Thus you may be measuring for a long time; however, it will become a habit, and it really doesn't take that much extra time.

- When you go to fast food establishments, don't get the super-duper portion when making your selections. Just because they ask doesn't mean you have to order the mammoth bucket o' fries. Stick with smallest portions available. Usually in fast food restaurants this is equal to a regular children's meal. If you don't have children, give the toy to any child you know.

- At a sit-down restaurant, if presented with "hearty" portions, eat only half of what is given to you. Have your server provide you with take out container and put away half of the meal to take home for your next meal. Do this even before you start eating if you know you will polish off the entire meal if you're not careful. If the meal has a half order option, then get the smaller size. The more food you are presented with, the more food you will eat.

- Split meals with a friend. If you go to a burger joint, split the fries, even if they are small. If you want dessert, go for it. Select something you can share with others.

- Order an appetizer as your main course. For example, many restaurants offer side salads in appetizer or main meal options, or allow you to order chicken, beef, or fish for an additional fee to round out the meal.

- Fool your eyes. When serving your meals, use smaller plates. Get used to using the salad plate as the dish you use for your main meals. This will fool your eyes into thinking there's more food than there actually is and leave you more satisfied.

Week 3 Let the Roughage Begin: A Word about Vegetables

So how is it going so far? Have you stuck to the food journal? Have you written down everything that you have been eating, including that one bite you had off your friend's dinner plate?

<u>By now you should be</u>:

- Writing everything you eat in your food journal.

- Drinking eight to twelve glasses of water/ fluid every day.

- Exercising for thirty minutes three to five days every week, working up to doing it on most days of the week.
    - *You can give your body a break in between sessions.*

- Measuring out portion sizes.

Now it is time to embark on Week 3. After reading the table of contents in this book, you may have dreaded reading this section of the book. You may have skimmed through it or skipped it altogether. I am hoping that you are now reading it to its entirety. This week I want you to have at least three to five servings of non-starchy vegetables every day. If you aren't eating any vegetables right now, start by have at least two each day and work up to having one to two servings per meal. You can eat more than three per day if you would like. This is one of the food groups where you can go overboard.

Vegetables are a freebie in my book (except for the starchy ones like potatoes and corn). As a general recommendation, one serving equals approximately half a cup cooked or one cup of raw vegetables. Again, I am sorry to report, starchy vegetables like potatoes and corn don't count here. Now, I'm not saying that you can't eat starchy vegetables; they just count in a different grouping in this book. Not to worry, the starchy vegetables have their place in the meal plan, and I will make sure to add them in (I do love my share of potatoes, in any form, I may add).

Why eat vegetables? They are a good source of essential vitamins, minerals, antioxidants, and fiber. Beans, technically a vegetable, albeit a starchy vegetable, are also an excellent source of protein, potassium, folic acid, iron, and magnesium. Look for more information on beans in Week 5 (Make the Switch to Whole Grains and Starches: What Does That Really Mean?) and Week 6 (Protein: The Building Blocks). Also, vegetables are low in calories and fat (at least most of them) while providing the body with much needed fuel. Finally, they may help protect you from chronic diseases such as various types of cancer, cardiovascular disease, obesity, and diabetes.

Tips:

- Stir-fry in low sodium broths, juices, or a small amount of flavored oil such as garlic flavored olive oil.

- Dip fresh cut vegetables with reduced fat or fat-free dressing (and do stick to the suggested serving size).

- Have a vegetable based soup at the start of a meal, or eat a garden salad with all vegetables with a low-fat or nonfat dressing (and stick to serving sizes).
- When at home you can have your soup or salad while you are preparing meals to prevent you from picking while you cook, and decrease your appetite for dinner. They don't call it "filler" for nothing!

- Dress up your omelets with onions, peppers, mushrooms, shredded carrots, broccoli, or squash.

- Sneak vegetables into pasta, casseroles, on top of pizza, in sandwiches, and in homemade salsas.

- Have a vegetable-based burger instead of a regular hamburger and top with lettuce, tomatoes, and onions.

- Mixed sautéed carrots, red peppers, onions, and garlic with ground sirloin for burgers and meatloaf.

- Have a sandwich of roasted vegetables instead of deli meats.

- Vary your vegetables, by varying the colors you consume. Each color vegetable represents different vitamins the vegetable is rich in.

- Use fresh, frozen or canned. When using frozen, make sure there aren't any added sauces. When buying canned, look for lower sodium choices and rinse through a strainer prior to using.

- Track the amount of vegetables you eat in your food log (see table 4).

Examples of one serving of vegetables:[6]

- 2 cups of raw kale (1 cup cooked)

- 1 cup cooked spinach

- 2 stalks of celery

- 2 medium carrots, or 3 ounces baby carrots (about 12)

- 10 broccoli florets (raw)

Table 4: Updated Journal   Date:_____

Table 4: Updated Journal   Date:_____

Breakfast Time:_____	Snack 1 Time:_____
_____ _____ _____ _____	_____ _____ _____
Lunch Time:_____	Snack 2 Time:_____
_____ _____ _____ _____	_____ _____ _____
Dinner Time:_____	Snack 3 Time:_____
_____ _____ _____ _____	_____ _____ _____
Exercise: _____ _____ _____ _____	Water Consumed: ☐☐☐☐ ☐☐☐☐ ☐☐☐☐ Other Beverages: _____ _____
Shopping List: _____ _____ _____ _____	Vegetables: ☐☐☐☐☐ Comments: _____ _____

63

Week 4 Fruit: Nature's Dessert

By now you should be:

- Writing everything you eat in your food journal.

- Drinking eight to twelve glasses of water/ fluid every day.

- Exercising for thirty minutes three to five days every week working up to doing it on most days of the week.
  - *You can give your body a break in between sessions.*

- Measuring out portion sizes.

- Consuming three to five or more servings of non-starchy vegetables each day.

For Week 4, I want you to incorporate two to four servings of fruit in each day. If you aren't eating any fruits right now, start by have at least one each day and work up to having one serving per meal or as a snack.

Why eat fruits? Mainly, you want to do it for many of the same benefits as consuming more vegetables. Increasing fruits in your meal plan can also dress up a meal and make it more appetizing by adding interesting flavors.

Tips
- Try various kinds of fruits that change with the seasons.

- Join your local food cooperatives (check the references section for a example Internet site).[7]

- Try various colors to ensure a varied nutrient intake.

- Try new fruits you haven't tried before and vary your intake with the changes in season. Try ugli, kiwis, pomegranate, or star fruit.

- Mix into hot and cold cereals for a sweeter flavor without adding extra sugar.

- Mix with fresh or frozen nonfat yogurt.

- Fruits make great desserts. Make them the main attraction for dessert with low-fat or nonfat whipped topping or yogurt (or with nonfat pudding for a twist).

- Have a smoothie made with fresh or frozen fruit (Check out Part III: Sample Menus: Main Meals and Snacks). When using frozen fruit, make sure it doesn't have any extra sauces or sugar added, and please, don't use frozen pulp; it is essential sugar with some added fruit for color and flavor.

- Combine with sugar-free gelatin (Check out Part III: Sample Menus: Main Meals and Snacks).

- Add fresh fruits to salads for a flavor twist.

- Track the amount of fruits you eat in your food log along with vegetables (see table 5).

<u>One serving equals approximately</u>:[8]

- 1 small to medium fruit (4 ounces)

- ½ of a large banana or 1 small banana

- 1¼ cup whole strawberries

- 2 small or 1 large plum (about 5 ounces total)

- 1 kiwi (3½ ounces total)

- 1 cup cubed papaya (8 ounces total)

- ½ cup cubed mango (5½ ounces total)

- ¾ cup cubed pineapple

- ½ cup of canned
    - *Look for varieties that are in unsweetened liquids or syrups*

- 4 ounces of juice (depending on the kind of juice)
    - *Remember, fruit juice usually has a very small amount of fiber and may have more calories than the fruit. Also, the fruit will fill you up more than the juice.*

- 2 tablespoons dried fruit

Table 5: Updated Journal   Date:_____

Table 5: Updated Journal   Date:_____

Breakfast Time:_____	Snack 1 Time:_____
_____ _____ _____ _____	_____ _____ _____ _____
Lunch Time:_____	Snack 2 Time:_____
_____ _____ _____ _____	_____ _____ _____ _____
Dinner Time:_____	Snack 3 Time:_____
_____ _____ _____ _____	_____ _____ _____ _____
Exercise: _____ _____ _____ _____	Water Consumed: ☐☐☐☐ ☐☐☐☐ ☐☐☐☐ Other Beverages: _____ _____
Shopping List: _____ _____ _____ _____	Vegetables: ☐☐☐☐☐ Fruits: ☐☐☐☐ Comments: _____ _____

Week 5 Make the Switch to Whole Grains and Starches (Including Starchy Vegetables): What Does That Really Mean?

By now you should be:

- Writing everything you eat in your food journal.

- Drinking eight to twelve glasses of water/ fluid every day.

- Exercising for thirty minutes three to five days every week working up to doing it on most days of the week.
  - *You can give your body a break in between sessions.*

- Measuring out portion sizes.

- Consuming three to five or more servings of non-starchy vegetables each day.

- Consuming two to four servings of fruit each day.

The latest buzzword in the food industry is whole grains. Take a look at grocery shelves, and you will see an abundance of products touting that they contain whole grains. So what are they? Basically, products containing whole grains contain the whole form of the grain, such as wheat, corn, rice, oats, barley, and rye just to name a few. Consuming the whole grain means just that: you consume all three parts of the grain (the bran, endosperm, and germ), as opposed to consuming just one part. By consuming the whole grain, you consume more protein, fiber, and nutrients including phytochemicals and antioxidants, than you would with just refined grains (like plain white bread).[9] Also, when half of your grains come from whole grains, you can decrease your risks of heart disease, stroke, colon cancer, diabetes, and obesity. [10]

Now, this doesn't mean that by consuming whole grains you will not become obese or suddenly will lose tons of weight. There's much more to weight loss than making one change; however, consuming whole grains can help. Also, whole grains provide the body with much needed fuel to keep you moving. Whole grains provide needed carbohydrates that the muscles use during exercise and for the brain to function. So please, whatever you do, don't avoid carbohydrates to lose weight. There are much better ways to cut calories than giving up these vital foods.

As I stated above, consuming whole grains can increase your fiber intake depending on which grain you consume. There are two major types of fiber: soluble and insoluble. The truth is, fiber passes through the body undigested, especially insoluble fiber, hence the name. Soluble fibers form a gel when mixed with a liquid. The soluble fiber helps reduce cholesterol by binding some it in the digestive tract, which may decrease your risk of heart disease. Increasing your fiber intake can decrease the absorption of calories, since fiber is difficult to digest. Foods rich in soluble fiber may decrease the absorption of calories, especially calories coming from carbohydrate rich foods including fruits and vegetables. If the absorption of calories is delayed, this can help control blood sugar levels, which in turn can help decrease the risks associated with diabetes.

Now, this doesn't mean that all you need to do to control your blood sugars is have more fiber, but it can help you better manage blood sugars. Soluble fiber has the added benefit of adding bulk to food. This makes you feel full much more quickly than simple or refined sugars that have little to no fiber at all, simply because they take up more room. For many of you, this will become extremely helpful in controlling your appetite. The bulk that fiber provides takes up room in the digestive tract. It can take up to twenty minutes or more for the brain to tell you that it is full. Thus, fiber can help that time pass by making you hold off from having another plateful of food.

A word for those of you who have a difficult time going to the bathroom (having a bowel movement that is): having more insoluble fiber can help in that department as well, thanks to the bulk it adds. Words of caution, though: increase the amount of fiber-rich foods you consume slowly. If you've been having little to no fiber in your diet and suddenly start having the recommended amount of twenty to thirty-eight grams each day (five to ten grams of that should come from soluble fiber) you may be plagued with even more constipation (or diarrhea), bloating, cramping, and for some indigestion.[11]

Up until now you have been having fruits, vegetables, and are consuming eight to twelve cups of water each and every day. Make sure you continue to do that, and start by increasing your consumption of whole grains by one portion each day until you are at three to six (preferable closer to six) each and every day. Continuing to have plenty of water will help because fiber absorbs water; thus by having enough fluid in the diet, things don't get stuck, so to speak.

You may be thinking, "If fiber is so good for me, why don't I just buy a fiber supplement instead?" I am not a fan of popping pills. Stick to getting your fiber from food and not from a pill (unless otherwise directed by you health care provider). An oral supplement usually does not provide all of the various nutrients that food can provide.

So what to look for when shopping? For one, you can look for the Whole Grain Stamp when walking down the aisles in the supermarket shelves. There are two stamps available. The first stamp available ensures that there are at least 50 percent (or more) whole grains per serving in the product, and the second stamp ensures that 100 percent of whole grains are present.[12] Also, look for buzzwords such as whole wheat, whole barley, whole oats, or stone ground. When in doubt, check the list of ingredients. The first ingredient listed should contain the word *whole*. If not, you may be taking a gamble on how much of the whole grain is available in the product. Be wary of marketing gimmicks. If it says "seven grain" or "twelve grain" and whole grain is the second ingredient listed, there may be less than 30 percent whole grains in the product.

Finally, look for the health claim that "diets rich in whole grain foods, and other plant foods and low in total fat, saturated fat, and cholesterol may help reduce the risk of heart disease and certain cancers."[13] What this means is that a manufacturer of a product can, under the provisions of the Food and Drug Administration Modernization Act of 1997 (FDAMA), notify the FDA of a health claim "based on an authoritative statement from an appropriate federal agency or the National Academy of Sciences (NAS)."[13] If the FDA does not forbid the manufacturer from making the claim within 120 days of receiving the notification, then the manufacturer can make the health claim.

What to do to up your intake:

- Try to allow six to eleven servings per day of foods classified as starches (stick to portion sizes). For weight loss, try to stay at approximately six to seven servings per day. At least three of the six to seven servings should consist of 100 percent whole grains, but by all means aim for all six to seven to come from whole grains.
- Look for breads that have at least two to three grams of fiber per serving. For example, look for 100 percent whole-wheat bread.

- Choose brown rice over white rice.

- Try whole-wheat pasta, which can have six to eight grams of fiber per serving instead of plain pasta, which has one to two grams of fiber per serving.

- Look for breakfast cereals that have at least three or more grams of fiber per serving (i.e., oatmeal). When possible, look for cereals with five or more grams of fiber.

- Vary your grains. Try grains you wouldn't normally try like barley or bulgur wheat (i.e., tabbouleh) instead of rice for a side dish.

- Include beans into your meal plan. The recommendation made by the United States Department of Agriculture states that we should all be consuming three cups of beans every week.[14] That can be broken down into half a cup per day. Get out the dry measuring cup; it really isn't that much. Although the Food Guide Pyramid lists them in two groups, in this book they fall under three: vegetables, starch, and protein. Ah, yes, you will hear about beans in another section of this book. Check out Week 6 (Protein: The Building Blocks) for tips on how to vary beans in your diet.

- Decrease the amount of sugar-packed, processed foods you consume. For example, cut back on (but I am by no means saying eliminate):
  o Regular sodas
  o Candy
  o Cookies
  o Pastries
  o Cakes
  o Sugar coated cereals
  o Frozen desserts

- Track the amount of starches (including starchy vegetables) you eat in your food log along with fruits and vegetables (see table 6).

Serving sizes

All are approximate estimates:[15]

- ½ cup of any cooked cereal

- ¾-1 cup of ready to eat, unsweetened cereal (depends on the cereal, check the nutrition facts label)

- ⅓ cup cooked rice or pasta (or 1 ounce dry)

- 1 ounce of any whole-grain bread (usually about 1 slice of regular or 2 slices for light bread)

- ½ cup of any starchy vegetables (for example, beans, peas, lentils, corn, plantains, squash, or potatoes) after cooking

- 1 mini muffin (1 ounce in weight)

- 1 ounce of any snack food (for example, saltines, animal crackers, popcorn, pretzels, or rice cakes). Look for more bang for your buck. Look at the label for serving sizes. Choose products that have larger serving sizes for the same amount of calories.

Starchy vegetables:[15]

- ½ cup of cooked beans

- ½ cup of peas

- ½ cup of corn kernels

- 1 cup canned pumpkin (generally comes pureed), no sugar added

- 3 ounces (or ½ cup) of sweet potato (or boniato)

- 3 ounces (or ½ cup) of malanga

- ½ cup prepared plantains

Table 6: Updated Journal   Date:_____

Table 6: Updated Journal   Date:_____

Breakfast Time:_____	Snack 1 Time:_____
_____ _____ _____ _____	_____ _____ _____ _____
Lunch Time:_____	Snack 2 Time:_____
_____ _____ _____ _____	_____ _____ _____ _____
Dinner Time:_____	Snack 3 Time:_____
_____ _____ _____ _____	_____ _____ _____
Exercise: _____ _____ _____ _____	Water Consumed: ☐☐☐☐ ☐☐☐☐ ☐☐☐☐ Other Beverages: _____ _____
Shopping List: _____ _____ _____ _____ _____	Vegetables: ☐☐☐☐☐ Fruits: ☐☐☐☐ Starches: ☐☐☐☐☐☐☐☐☐☐ Comments:_____ _____

Week 6 Protein: The Building Blocks

<u>By now you should be</u>:

- Writing everything you eat in your food journal.

- Drinking eight to twelve glasses of water/ fluid every day.

- Exercising for thirty minutes three to five days every week working up to doing it on most days of the week.
  o *You can give your body a break in between sessions.*

- Measuring out portion sizes.

- Consuming three to five or more servings of non-starchy vegetables each day.

- Consuming two to four servings of fruit each day.

- Consuming three to six whole-grain-rich foods daily (six to eleven total servings per day of all foods classified as starches including starchy vegetables and whole grains).

High-protein "diets" have been all the rage in the last few years, and they made a powerful comeback when I first became a registered dietitian. Soon after completing my dietetic internship, I began my career at a small, community hospital working with predominately cardiology patients, many of which had just suffered from heart attacks and strokes. Many of the patients I encountered also suffered from diabetes and diabetes-related complications.

I can recall an incident that occurred during my employment there with a general physician (not a cardiologist) who worked within the hospital. The physician had recommended that his patient begin a high-protein, carbohydrate-free "diet" to bring down his blood sugars to control his diabetes and lose excess weight. He had ordered a nutrition consult for "diet" education on this prescribed diet.

A note to my readers:

When you are a patient in a hospital, registered dietitians are, in most institutions, bound by the "diet" order or prescription. If there is no diet order, then the department cannot send a tray no matter how many meals or days you have gone without eating. If you are a diabetic and receive regular sugar, check your meal ticket. If it says you are on a regular or general "diet", the nutrition department has no way of knowing that you are a diabetic and may send regular sugar instead of a nonnutritive sweetener. Thus, when a physician or other health care provider with privileges writes for nutrition education on a specific "diet," I am bound to that order, unless I find it to be inappropriate or totally incorrect.

I shall proceed. I found no reason for the patient in question to be on a high protein, carbohydrate free "diet" and contacted the doctor for an explanation. He happened to be in the hospital, so I waited. He explained that the plan worked for him, and he now recommends it to all his patients. Now just because a fad "diet" worked for him doesn't mean that this is proof for me to instruct patients to use this "diet" for diabetes management and/or weight loss. I follow an evidence-based practice, which just means that I base my career and my education of patients and clients on scientific evidence or proof. I offered to do just that and needless to say taught an appropriate meal plan based on the patient's needs.

When the high-protein diets made a comeback in recent years, you couldn't walk the supermarket shelves without seeing the plethora of high-protein, low-carbohydrate products. Any carbohydrate-rich product available had a low-carbohydrate substitute such as cereal, bread, yogurt, milk, snack bars, ice cream, and other desserts. Many people have lost weight following these plans; however, once off the plans the weight gain often comes right back. Some, mainly those using all the new low-carb products, didn't lose any weight, and some even gained some weight. Why, you may ask? Basically it boils down to what I have said before. A calorie is a calorie is a calorie. Those who lost weight following high protein "diets" did so mainly because they consumed less calories than their bodies need on a daily basis. Heck, when you eliminate carbohydrate rich foods, you are eliminating all fruits, juices, starches, starchy vegetables, and most dairy products. However, some gain weight, especially when they substitute carbohydrates with low-carbohydrate products. Usually these products have the exact amount of calories as the regular version, and sometimes more.

With all this talk about protein, you may be thinking that I think protein is a bad food. That's not it at all. Protein is an important part of your daily meal plan. It provides the body with fuel and contains the much-needed "building blocks" for your muscles, organs, and bones. Having enough protein will help boost your immune system in order to ward off diseases. Finally, protein builds and repairs tissues in the body. Although protein is important, many of us get plenty of it.

The goal for this week is to start to choose lower fat protein sources to reduce fat, cholesterol, and calories. Fat has more calories per gram than carbohydrates and protein. By choosing lower fat protein sources, you will be cutting back on excess calories in your meal plan.

Preferably, try to have some protein with each meal and snack. Protein as part of a healthy meal plan can help keep you full. Since it takes longer to digest, having protein with meals can help keep you full for longer than if you missed it with the meal, curbing your hunger. Make sure to have at least two to three servings each day, or six to nine ounces total in the day. For every ounce you have, check off a circle on your food journal.

What to choose:

- Look for beef with little to no marbling (the fatty streaks in the meat) and with little fat surrounding the meat. If present, cut fat surrounding meat prior to cooking.

- Look for the words *round, sirloin,* and *tenderloin*. For example: pork tenderloin, top/bottom round, sirloin, or flank steaks. Avoid prime cuts. Yes, these are quite tasty, but calorie wise you will pay the price. And yes, fat does give food more flavor; however, there are other ways of increasing flavor in your meals while allowing you to cut out the fat. Save the higher fat meats for special occasions only.

- Use 90-95 percent lean ground beef, pork, chicken, or turkey. Or try veggie ground (looks like ground beef and is used to replace ground beef in popular recipes). When using veggie grounds remember that they are not calorie free; however, they often have less calories and definitely less fat than animal products (and are cholesterol free).

- Try to switch to a low-fat bacon such as turkey bacon (please read labels), lean/low-salt ham, or Canadian bacon, or even try soy-based breakfast "sausages" and soy-based "bacon."

- Do you have a hankering for some hot dogs right off the grill? Try reduced-fat or fat-free beef, chicken, or turkey franks. Often, the lower fat versions also have less salt. You can even find vegetarian hot dogs (usually made of soy) for a change of pace. These tend to be low in fat and cholesterol free.

- When eating poultry, choose the white meat over the dark meat to decrease fat and calories. Go one step further and take the skin off before you cook the bird so you are not tempted to eat the skin later. If you want to keep the skin on during cooking to lock in the moisture, make sure you take it off before you put it on your plate if you know you will be tempted to eat it afterwards.

- Choose low-fat deli meats. Also, when at the deli counter, try to choose the lower salt varieties. Avoid heavily processed meats like salami or bologna. Some manufactures make low-fat or nonfat processed versions, but make sure to watch the salt content for those of you who need to watch your salt intake.

- Increase your seafood consumption. There is more to seafood than just frozen fish sticks. Now, don't get me wrong; you don't have to buy only fresh seafood. Just avoid frozen products that have been breaded and fried prior to packaging, and be careful of products that have evidence of freezer burn or appear to be thawing out. Seafood provides an excellent source of protein, is low in saturated fat (the "bad" fat), and many varieties are rich in omega-3 fatty acids. Increasing your consumption of seafood may keep you heart healthy and help in a child's growth and development.[16] Increase your consumption to two to three times per week by using seafood to replace meats or poultry products in many of your favorite dishes. Vary your intake by trying seafood that you have never eaten before like codfish, flounder, salmon, fresh tuna (or canned in water, not oil), haddock, halibut, trout, and red snapper. Avoid deep fat frying and stick to steaming, baking, broiling, or sautéing in a small amount of oil such as olive or canola oil. Most seafood cooks in less than ten minutes or so, making it easy to enjoy any night of the week.

- Try egg white omelets or try using an egg substitute. Limit your consumption of egg yolks. Each egg has only 75 calories and 5 grams of fat, but about 213 milligrams of cholesterol.[17] Each egg white has only 17 calories, no fat or cholesterol.[17] Allow yourself three to four whole eggs a week; just watch how you cook them. If you use egg whites have as many as you want; however, please don't throw the yolks away. Save them and use them in other recipes, or just buy prepackaged egg whites.

- Limit consumption of organ meats (i.e., liver). Some, like kidneys, are low in fat but still high in cholesterol.

- Try to incorporate vegetarian protein sources such as tofu or soy-based replacements. Add tofu to your favorite stews and casseroles to cut fat, cholesterol, calories, and dollars spent. There are numerous options these days to allow for variety, and there are many recipes out there in order to make your own. Soy-based products tend to be low in fat, cholesterol free, and cheaper than their animal-based versions.[18] Also, many are also excellent sources of fiber.

- Use quinoa instead of your usual starch. As opposed to wheat, it has a higher percentage of protein and is also a great source of fiber. Unlike most grains, it contains a balanced set of essential amino acids, making it great for vegetarians or those of you just trying to cut back on the amount of animal foods consumed.

- Cooked beans, peas, and lentils. Yes, folks, beans again. You may remember them from a previous week's tips. Beans, peas, and lentils are great because they provide starch (for energy), fiber, and protein without adding a whole lot of fat. Also, they have no saturated fat, cholesterol, or salt (unless you use the canned variety). When using canned beans, rinse them off first in a strainer to remove some of the added salt. Finally, they are cheap. One can of beans usually costs less than one dollar (even less if you wait for a sale), and unlike most meats, you can usually cut coupons for beans. When choosing beans, check off one starch as well as one protein on your food journal. Ways to increase beans in your meal plan:

- o Buy several kinds of canned beans (unless you prepare yourself) and rinse out prior to using.
- o Throw half a cup per serving into soups, salads, stews, and casseroles. Chances are you won't even taste that they are in there.
- o Have bean-based soups as a main meal at least once a week topped with one ounce of cheese and a serving of reduced-fat sour cream.
- o Have over rice or plain as a side dish.
- o Make homemade salsa with black beans (Check out Part III: Sample Days for a sample recipe).

- Try roasted nuts (high in fat but from a vegetable source). Try to stick to the unsalted variety. Make sure to stick with portion sizes since nuts are a concentrated source of fat and calories.

- Use peanut butter or any other nut butter as a spread for things like wheat toast or whole-grain waffles instead of butter or margarine.

- Sunflower seeds (high in fat, however, the good kind). Try some in salads or just grab a serving to snack on. Again watch the serving sizes.

Serving sizes

All are approximate estimates:

- ½ cup cooked bean, peas, or lentils. Be especially careful when adding beans to your meal plan. This is one of those foods that can cause some damage if you start by consuming too large of a serving. For some people, consuming beans can cause some gastrointestinal discomfort. Your body will adjust if you eat them consistently so that eventually you will not have gassiness. Start with ¼ cup each day and work your way up to ½ cup.

- 3 ounces cooked poultry, seafood, or beef (about 4 ounces before you cook it). For every ounce that you have, mark off one of the circles on the food journal. Many books and magazines will tell you this is about the size of a deck of cards. That really isn't that big. Most people consume much more than the suggested serving size, and this is where the calories add up. Mark off three circles in your food journal.

- 1 egg or 2 egg whites

- 1 ounce of nuts

- 1 ounce of seeds such as pumpkin, sunflower, or flaxseed

Table 7: Updated Journal   Date:_____

Table 7: Updated Journal   Date:_____

Breakfast Time:_____	Snack 1 Time:_____
Lunch Time:_____	Snack 2 Time:_____
Dinner Time:_____	Snack 3 Time:_____
Exercise: _____ _____ _____ _____	Water Consumed: ☐☐☐☐ ☐☐☐☐ ☐☐☐☐ Other Beverages: _____ _____
Shopping List:_____ _____ Comments:_____ _____	Vegetables: ☐☐☐☐☐ Fruits: ☐☐☐☐ Starches: ☐☐☐☐☐☐☐☐☐☐ Protein: ☐☐☐☐☐☐☐☐

Week 7 Milk, Cheese, and Yogurt (Dairy)

By now you should be:

- Writing everything you eat in your food journal.

- Drinking eight to twelve glasses of water/ fluid every day.

- Exercising for thirty minutes three to five days every week working up to doing it on most days of the week.
  - *You can give your body a break in between sessions.*

- Measuring out portion sizes.

- Consuming three to five or more servings of non-starchy vegetables each day.

- Consuming two to four servings of fruit each day.

- Consuming three to six whole-grain-rich foods daily (six to eleven total servings per day of all foods classified as starches including starchy vegetables and whole grains).

- Consuming two to three servings of protein-rich foods each day (or six to nine ounces total in the day).

This week you embark on choosing three servings per day of choose low-fat or nonfat dairy products (milk, cheeses, and yogurt). All three groups are also good sources of protein; however, for now mark off a dairy on your food journal when consuming (more on that when we get to meal spacing).

- *Note for those of you who are lactose intolerant: choose lactose-free products like cheese, milk, yogurt, ice cream, or use products that allow you to digest dairy products.*

- *Note for those of you who are allergic to dairy products: talk to your health care provider or better yet a registered dietitian about other sources of calcium or a calcium supplement. You can also supplement by using products that use fortified soy milk (or other fortified substitute) instead of traditional cow's milk.*

There are many reasons to have dairy products in your meal plan. Not only does it provide some protein, it is an excellent source of calcium. People who consume at least three servings per day of calcium, especially from dairy sources, are more likely to lose weight when combined with a reduced-calorie meal plan.

Dairy products are important in:[19]

- Maintaining bone structure/bone mass, preventing osteoporosis.

- Muscle contraction/relaxation.

- The function of nerves, blood clotting and blood pressure, and immune defenses.

- Possibly decreasing your chances of colon cancer.

- Possibly decreasing the symptoms of PMS.

- Benefits associated with important nutrients including calcium, potassium, magnesium, and vitamin A.

One drawback to having dairy products in the diet is the fat and cholesterol content of full-fat products. However, by choosing low- and nonfat sources, you significantly lower fat and cholesterol, as well as cut calories from your meal plan.

Choose:

- Skim or 1% milk.

- Reduced-fat or nonfat cheeses (including cheeses like cottage cheese and ricotta cheese).

- Low-fat or nonfat yogurt.

- For dessert, fat-free pudding or low-fat (or fat-free) ice cream or frozen yogurt.

Serving sizes

All are approximate estimates:

- 1 ounce of cheese.[20] I must admit that I have a weakness for cheese. I have not met a variety that I haven't absolutely loved. Instead of giving it up altogether, I stick with the regular variety and make sure I measure out my portions. One great trick is to stick with strong flavors like extra sharp, Monterey Jack, blue, or freshly grated Parmesan cheeses. Due to their strong flavors, a small amount goes a long way. If you try the low-fat varieties and love them, then go ahead and substitute them for the regular versions.

- 1 cup (8 ounces) skim milk or 1% milk.[20] Skim milk contains 80 calories and zero fat per serving, and 1% contains 110 calories and 2.5 grams of fat per serving. Many patients have told me in the past that they have switched from whole milk to 2% milk. Whole milk contains 150 calories and 8 grams of fat per serving, and switching to 2% is better because it has 130 calories and 5 grams of fat per serving. While I applaud people for making changes in the right direction, I encourage them to continue to cut back until they reach skim milk.

- ½ cup evaporated milk.[20] Try to stick with skim or 1% varieties.

- ⅓ cup dry skim milk powder. Make sure you have a clean water supply before reconstituting.

- 1 cup (8 ounces) of nonfat or low-fat yogurt (however, many varieties come in 6-ounce containers). When shopping for yogurt, keep in mind that all yogurts are not made alike. Regular, plain yogurt has approximately 180 calories and 9 grams of fat per serving. Flavored, regular yogurt usually has additional calories (usually, mostly from sugar). Low-fat, plain yogurt has approximately 120 calories and 2 grams of fat per serving. Again, flavored yogurt usually has up to 100 additional calories. Fat-free, plain yogurt has approximately 100 calories and zero fat per serving. Unfortunately, again flavored yogurt will add more unwanted calories. So are you doomed to have only plain, fat-free yogurt? Not at all. You can flavor it by blending in a serving of fresh or fresh frozen fruit (not frozen pulp, which has additional calories). If added sweetness is your desire, use a nonnutritive, calorie-free sweetener. You could use maple syrup or honey, but watch your serving sizes and make sure to mark off a starch as well as a dairy off your food journal. Short on time, and unable to blend your own? Then choose light yogurt. It usually has approximately 60-80 calories and zero fat per serving (depending on the brand you choose).

- ¼ cup reduced-fat or nonfat cottage cheese. Whole-fat cottage cheese has approximately 120 calories and 5 grams of fat per serving [21], while 2% has about 90 calories and 2.5 grams of fat per serving.[22] You can go further by going all the way down to fat free, but if it doesn't taste good to you then stick with the 2%. All have about 12 grams of protein, making them excellent choices of added protein, as well as much needed calcium. Have with your morning toast instead of eggs topped with some cinnamon and a packet of sugar or nonnutritive sweetener, mix fat-free cottage cheese with fat-free ricotta cheese for added texture, or have with a cup of sliced fresh fruit as a snack.

- ¼ cup (or 2 ounces) of ricotta cheese.[20] You can get it as full fat, low fat, or nonfat. For most recipes you can get away with using low fat. When using the nonfat variety, consider the suggestion listed above by supplementing half the desired quantity with fat-free cottage cheese instead for added texture. Mix with pasta to give sauces an added creaminess without adding as much fat as heavy cream would.

Table 8: Updated Journal   Date:_____

Breakfast Time:_____	Snack 1 Time:_____
_____ _____ _____ _____	_____ _____ _____ _____
Lunch Time:_____	Snack 2 Time:_____
_____ _____ _____ _____ ____	_____ _____ _____ _____ ____
Dinner Time:_____	Snack 3 Time:_____
_____ _____ _____ _____	_____ _____ _____ _____
Exercise: _____ _____ _____ _____	Water Consumed: ☐☐☐☐ ☐☐☐☐ ☐☐☐☐ Other Beverages: _____ _____
Shopping List:_____ _____ Comments:_____ _____	Vegetables: ☐☐☐☐☐ Fruits: ☐☐☐☐ Starches: ☐☐☐☐☐☐☐☐☐☐ Protein: ☐☐☐☐☐☐☐☐☐ Dairy: ☐☐☐

Week 8 Fat: It Has Gotten a Bad Rap

Have you been told by your health care provider that your cholesterol is high and you need to lower your fat intake? Do you know what that exactly means? Over the years the verdict on fat in the diet has been cloudy at best. For many years fat and fatty foods have been labeled as "bad" and forbidden from the diet. As discussed earlier, we as a society even went through a fat-free "diet" craze, often going wild for the latest foods that promised to be fat free and good for you. Unfortunately, fat-free diets did not work, and obesity continued to rise to overwhelming rates.

Reducing the amount of total fat that you are consuming can be tricky. With all the new labels out there, it's hard to know what any of them mean. Many products carry labels touting that they are low fat, reduced fat, nonfat, light (or lite), or that they contain no trans fats. What do they all mean? Luckily there are rules in the labeling game. If you are unsure, compare products to one another when you are in the supermarket. Check out table 9 for what certain words on a label mean.

Table 9: Reading Labels

Label Claim	What it means
Low Calorie	Product contains less than or equal to 40 calories per serving.
Light (or Lite)	This term can be applied to calories and fat. If a label says light (or lite) it means it has either ⅓ less calories than the regular version or at least 50% less fat than its regular counterpart.
Calorie Free	Less than or equal to 5 calories per serving.
Reduced	This term can be applied to calories, total fat, saturated fat, cholesterol, or sodium. It basically means that the product has less than 25% compared to the regular version.
Low Fat	Less than or equal to 3 grams of fat per serving.
Low Saturated Fat	Less than or qual to 1 gram of saturated fat per serving.
Nonfat	Less than or equal to ½ gram of total fat per serving.
Trans Fat Free	Less than 0.5 gram per serving.

So now that you know what certain words on packages mean, how much fat should you be consuming? I must note that I am not expecting you to follow a fat-free meal plan. Do not completely eliminate fat from your meals and snacks! You actually need fat in your daily meal plan for your body to function at its peak performance. Although too much of it is not a good thing, especially since it is a concentrated calorie provider containing nine calories per gram of fat, it does provide essential nutrients that the body can't make on its own. Fat is a nutrient that the body uses for other functions like the production of cell membranes and in several hormone-like compounds that can actually regulate your blood pressure and heart rate. Also, you need fat to carry fat-soluble vitamins in the body like A, D, E, and K.

Fat in the body also provides a layer of protection from the cold by being the insulation for the body and helps by providing a layer of protection for your internal organs (like built-in shock absorbers). However, too thick of a layer is not good (remember, too much of a good thing is not always good!). Finally, fat assists in giving your hair and skin a healthy glow that so many pay hundred of dollars for in expensive creams and moisturizers.

Besides being necessary for your body to function correctly, fat really does make foods taste better by enhancing the flavor and increasing the level of moistness to a dish. Also, using a small amount of fat can make it easier to cook. (Have you ever tried to use nonfat butter when frying up an egg? If you haven't, please don't because it will burn.) Ice cream just tastes better when it is made with heavy cream. Also, fat helps you feel full after a meal; it curbs your appetite since it is more calorie dense than foods that lack it, and it takes quite a while to digest.

Please read that last sentence twice. Although it can help make you feel full, since it is calorie dense, eating too much of it can lead you to consume too many calories and hinder weight-loss efforts. Remember, a calorie is a calorie is a calorie no matter where it comes from. Eat too many, you gain weight. Eat too little, you lose weight. There is a happy medium.

There is a way to decrease the amount of total fat you eat, lose weight, and still enjoy foods. The technical recommendation for fat intake based on the "Dietary Guidelines for Americans 2005" is to "keep total fat intake between 20 to 35 percent of calories, with most fats coming from sources of polyunsaturated and monounsaturated fatty acids, such as fish, nuts, and vegetable oils" and to "consume less than 10 percent of calories from saturated fatty acids and less than three hundred milligrams per day of cholesterol, and keep trans fatty acid consumption as low as possible."[23] Huh? No wonder the public is so confused.

When you check out the fat section of a nutrition label on a product, the first thing listed is the total fat, followed by a breakdown of the fats, which can include saturated, polyunsaturated, monounsaturated, and since January of 2006 also must list if it contains trans fats and how much. Also, food labels also tell you how much cholesterol an item contains. Basically, anything of animal origin will contain some level of cholesterol, including all kinds of meat, poultry, seafood, eggs, and milk products. Anything plant based including starches, fruits, and vegetables will not. This does not mean that they are fat free, only cholesterol free. For example, avocados and nuts contain fat; however, do not contain any cholesterol.

Your body makes all of the cholesterol it needs, so unless you're an infant, you really don't need any in your meals or snacks. Now, to completely avoid cholesterol you would have to completely avoid all animal products. I don't expect you to entirely remove animal products from your meal plan, just to make some adjustments and cut back a bit. If you want to completely give them up, then go for it (however, I do recommend that you seek out a registered dietitian to help ensure that you have a balanced menu).

Not all fats are created equal, and some are better for you than others. Having too much of the "bad fats" can increase your cholesterol levels and increase your likelihood of coronary artery disease. The offenders are saturated and trans fatty acids causing increases in cholesterol levels in the blood (especially LDL cholesterol), even more than the cholesterol in the foods you eat. Trans fatty acids can also decrease levels of the good cholesterol (HDL) that help decrease a person's risk of coronary artery disease. Saturated fats are found, like cholesterol, mostly in animal-based foods; however, unlike cholesterol there are some plant-based foods like coconut, palm, and some other tropical oils that contain saturated fat.

Trans fatty acids are for the most part are made, not born. They are born by the process of hydrogenation, which basically means adding hydrogen to vegetable oil, making the fat more solid. Trans fats are usually found in commercially prepared foods like cookies and cakes, and often used in many fast food establishments to fry foods such as donuts (yes, donuts are fried) and French fries. Since January 2006, many manufactures have eliminated them from their products because of the bad rap trans fatty acids have (and rightfully so). Although, I am grateful that trans fatty acids are being eliminated, this alone will not cause you to lose weight. Many of the foods that used to contain trans fat are still calorie rich and poor in total nutrition, so it is still best to use them in moderation.

So if the saturated and trans fats are the bad fats, are there any good fats? Of course there are. Remember, I mentioned that you do need some fat daily in your meal plan. The monounsaturated and polyunsaturated fats (which include the omega-3 fatty acids you have heard so much about and have probably seen so many foods fortified with) are considered the "good" fats. By replacing some of the bad offenders with the good fats, you can help reduce your bad cholesterol, also known as LDL cholesterol. The omega-3 fatty acids may also decrease your risk for coronary artery disease and can even help lower your blood pressure. [24] Every day research is coming out on other benefits of increasing your intake of omega-3 fatty acids, so keep an eye out. Omega-3 fatty acids are found mostly in fatty fish like salmon, lake trout, mackerel, albacore tuna, sardines, and herring; however, you can also find in them in flaxseeds, flaxseed oil, and walnuts. [24] Other polyunsaturated fats include vegetable oils (i.e. corn, soy, sunflower, safflower, and cottonseed). [24] Monounsaturated fats are found in avocados, most of the nuts and oils like olive, canola, and peanut oil. [24]

So now for the breakdown. Fat has more than double the calories (at 9 calories per gram) than carbohydrates and protein which come in at 4 calories per gram. For example, a glass of whole, full-fat milk has 150 calories per eight-ounce serving and 8 grams of fat. Thus 72 of the total 150 calories come from fat.

Two percent milk has 120 calories per eight-ounce serving and 5 grams of fat. So 45 calories of the total 120 calories come from fat. One percent milk has 100 calories per eight-ounce serving and 2.5 grams of fat. So approximately 23 calories of the total 100 calories are from fat. Finally, skim milk has 80 calories per eight-ounce serving and no fat.

Now, it doesn't seem like a lot of calories to cut, but if you drink three glasses of whole milk a day, you would be consuming 450 calories just through milk. By cutting back to 1% milk, you cut 150 calories daily and still get to enjoy what you're craving.

With that said here are some tips to help you cut back on your total fat, your consumption of "bad" fat, total cholesterol, and trans fats:

- Look for products that say they are low in fat and in calories.

- Get out the measuring spoons. Often you can use regular oils, butters, dressings, and condiments. Many of us just go overboard. Check the label and stick with the listed serving size, or have less than the suggested serving.

- When using oils, stick with canola, olive oil, peanut, sunflower, or soybean oil. Canola has the lowest amount of saturated fat and is a source of omega-3 fatty acids and works great for baking.

- Use flavored oils so that you can use a smaller amount, such as sesame or peanut oil. Also, infuse olive oil by soaking fresh herbs and spices to kick up the flavor. By adding more flavors to the oil, you can get away with using less oil, especially in salads and marinades.

- Bake, grill, broil, boil, barbecue, steam, stir-fry, microwave, or roast (with a drip pan).

- Use nonstick cookware, often eliminating the need for added oils and/or butters.

- Use herbs and spices to flavor foods. Just because you are cutting down on your fat consumption doesn't mean that your meals can't be full of flavor. Please, whatever you do, don't add salt to your meals because you cut the fat. Try dried or fresh rosemary, allspice, basil, caraway seeds, chives, curry powder, garlic powder, marjoram, mint, onion powder, oregano, paprika, pimiento, sage, and/or sesame seeds. When using high-sodium condiments like soy sauce, use so sparingly (a little goes a long way) and opt for the lower sodium versions when available.

- Avoid eating fried foods.

- Try baked potato chips or fat-free potato chips and snacks.

- Try baked French fries.

- Try baked chicken (or any other fried food) versus fried using crushed bran flakes for breading.

- Use regular or low-salt chicken, beef, or vegetable broth instead of butter or margarine when making mashed potatoes and sautéing vegetables.

- Use cooking sprays or chicken, beef, or vegetable broths instead of oils when broiling or sautéing meats, poultry, and seafood.

- Use low-fat mayonnaise, mustard, ketchup relish, or barbecue sauce for condiments (make sure to watch your portion sizes).

- Use reduced-fat or fat-free salad dressings and gravies. Make sure to stick to serving sizes because these calories can add up very quickly.

- Choose reduced-fat or nonfat cream cheese (or try Neufchatel cheese), sour cream, and cottage cheeses.

- Marinate meats in nonfat marinades to increase flavor without adding fat.

- Top your burger with sliced avocado instead of sliced cheese. Make sure to stick with portion sizes.

- Use whipped or reduced-fat butter or choose margarine instead. Remember, regular butter is high in saturated fat and contains cholesterol (made from the fat from cow's milk). Margarine is a better choice because it is made from vegetable based oils; however, some may contain trans fats. Now that is the technical recommendation. Whether you choose regular butter or margarine, they both have similar amounts of total fat and calories. Remember: a calorie is a calorie is a calorie. Watch your serving sizes, reduce the total amount you consume, and if possible choose the lower fat versions.

- Have clear broth soups instead cream soups (unless the cream soup is a low-fat version).

Serving sizes (for fats only)

All are approximate estimates (based on common labels):

- 1 tablespoon butter or margarine (try to use 1 teaspoon).

- 1 tablespoon of most oils (try to use 1 teaspoon).

- Salad dressing (regular/full fat): 1-2 tablespoons

PART II:
Implementing What You Have Learned

Grocery Shopping

So for approximately eight weeks or so you have learned the basics and laid down the groundwork for changing your daily habits when it comes to food and physical fitness. Now you will begin to learn how to put a plan in place and into action by mapping out your daily meals. Planning your meals on a daily basis will ensure that you stay on course with your goals and help you avoid straying too far off your new selected path.

Planning is especially important when eating away from home, while on vacation, a business trip, or at a restaurant, social gathering, family affair, professional function, or any other function where food takes center stage. Also, having an idea of what you will be eating ahead of time will help prevent you from consuming foods you normally wouldn't eat or don't even like.

Getting the Groceries

Have you ever gone to the supermarket without a list of what you need to buy? Sure you have; we all have done it. Well, at least many of you have done this at one time or another. Many of you may hit the markets each and every time without a list. Going without a list is the wrong course of action. For one thing, you will probably be there twice as long. Whenever I forget my list, I find myself wandering from aisle to aisle to make sure that I don't forget anything. It never fails. As soon as I get home, I realize that I forgot a crucial thing like soy milk (can't have my morning cup of java without my vanilla soy milk). Going from aisle to aisle is fine when I am checking out a new supermarket or specialty food store like gourmet shops, but not for the everyday shopping. Most of us just don't have the luxury of time to do it.

Whether you are going to a large supermarket, wholesale club, or local corner store, having a list of items you need to purchase will save time, money, and most importantly prevent you from purchasing pricey impulse items you don't really want and definitely don't need. Impulse items in the supermarket can include food (i.e., candy, chocolate, and soda) as well as non-food items such as magazines and toys.

To prevent spending excess money and bringing home unwanted bags of groceries, make sure to leave your house prepared. Head out to the office supply store, or any store that carries stationary, and purchase a pad with a magnet on the back of it and place on your refrigerator door. Stainless steel appliances in your kitchen? Then designate a spot on the counter, or buy a bulletin or fabric board and put the pad there. If you have a computer in your kitchen or prefer to use your electronic organizer or phone, then set up a file in there for your food shopping list. Just make sure that you have quick access to it, or set it up and print it out and place on the refrigerator or bulletin board. Every time you run out of something, put it on your list. Every time you decide you want to try a new recipe, write the ingredients you need on the list. Sure, you could just tear it out of the magazine or bring the whole cookbook with you when you go food shopping, but that defeats the purpose of the list. The list is meant to simplify your life, streamline your shopping experience, and maximize your time.

If you're anything like me, you buy many of your items using discounted coupons and purchase predominately sale items. I remember as a little girl watching my mother open up the Sunday newspapers, cutting the coupons and circling items in the local supermarket circulars. When we would get to the store, she would hand me a few coupons and a small shopping basket and instruct me to get only what was on the coupons. If I came back with anything that was not on a coupon, it went right back on the shelf. I swore up in down (in my mind) I would never do the same. Here I am, over twenty years later, doing the exact same thing, although my mother has it down to a science, and I am not nearly as good at the savings as she is. However, I aspire to be there someday.

So along with your list, check circulars and coupons before hitting the market. On Sunday mornings clip all the coupons that you are going to clip. Try to organize them by departments in the supermarket, and pull out any that you will be using that day and keep them together with your list. Once you get to the market, take out your list and your coupons, and attack. Try to stick to only what is on your list and nothing else. Avoid the chocolate-covered cupcakes that are a dollar a box, unless they were on your list (but more on that later).

The majority of the staples you need will be located on the perimeter of the store. The others like cereals, canned goods, condiments, etc., will be located in the aisles in between. When you get to the checkout counter or cashier, try to overlook the tasty treats that are awaiting you.

When you get home from the supermarket, set some time aside to wash, cut up, and chop all of the fruits and vegetables so that they are quickly available for snacks, and your favorite recipes. Also, remember to put away the perishables in the refrigerator or freezer.

SPECIAL NOTE

Before you head out the door to grocery shop, make yourself a meal or have a snack. The worst thing you can do when grocery shopping is getting there when you are starving. When you go food shopping on an empty stomach, you may buy foods that you normally wouldn't eat or are trying to avoid, like the chocolate-covered cupcakes. When hunger strikes, everything you see will look tasty, especially the foods you have a weakness for. Do yourself a favor and have some carrot sticks or a sandwich before you leave the house.

To recap:

- Create a running shopping list.

- Cut your coupons every week.

- Check the circulars for your local supermarkets.

- If using coupons, group your list with the coupons you are using.

- Have a meal or snack right before heading out to the market.

Meal Spacing: This Isn't a Starvation Plan

I have discussed in detail the importance of "a calorie is a calorie is a calorie," and I'm sure that you are sick of hearing about it. Just when you thought you'd read all you needed to know about it, you are about to read a little more. Each and every person's metabolism is different. Your body needs a certain amount of calories to function. You need calories for everything from your heart beating to blinking your eyes. The more active a person you are, the more calories you burn, the more calories you will need to consume in order to function on a daily basis. The less active a person you are, the lower the amount of calories you will need to consume in order to function on a daily basis.

There is such a thing as lowering and increasing your metabolism. You may have previously thought to cut out a meal or two here and there to save yourself some excess calories. When you starve yourself on a regular basis, your body begins the process of adjusting to that calorie level. The body goes into survival mode. For example, let's say you were eating two thousand calories each day and then gradually (or drastically) go down to one thousand calories per day. You would initially lose weight; however, at some point, your body will eventually compensate and learn to function and perform on the lesser amount of calories. So what happens when you go above one thousand calories? Your body latches on to the extra calories and stores them (since it no longer needs the excess anymore) and saves it for a later time. Think of it as your body preparing for hibernation. Yes, we have been over this earlier in the book; however I felt that it needed to be repeated.

So what have we learned? Don't starve yourself! This can put a stop to weight loss efforts or even make you gain weight. Try to keep the body constantly supplied with energy by eating small and frequent meals. Ideally, you want to eat about five or six times per day instead of three large meals. When you divvy up your daily meal into five or six meals, you keep the body constantly supplied with energy, which will prevent you from overeating since you will never really be hungry. Your body actually burns calories in order to digest the food that you eat, so ideally the more frequently you eat, the more you will burn. The key, however, is to have smaller portions at each meal, not consume five or six large meals.

Ground Rules

- As a rule of thumb, have at least two total servings of any carbohydrates—for example any whole grain, fruit, low-fat or nonfat milk, or yogurt—with every meal or snack. Milk and yogurt are classified as carbohydrates as wells as a dairy choice, however, in your food journal, check off a dairy choice and not a starch.
  - When snacking you can have one to two serving of the foods listed above.

- Vegetables (the non-starchy ones) are considered freebies in this plan, since most of us don't have enough of them.

- The majority of registered dietitians will tell you that starchy vegetables like potatoes, corn, or beans don't count as vegetables because they usually have as much carbohydrate and calories per serving as a one-ounce piece of bread. Starchy vegetables are healthy; however, because of their calorie and carbohydrate content, count them as a starch. Refer back to the whole grains section (and vegetable section for the starchy vegetables) for serving sizes and nutrition food labels.

- Have at least one ounce of protein with every meal or snack.

  o Protein-rich foods include meats, poultry, seafood, eggs, nuts (including peanut butter), cheeses (which can also count as a dairy), and soy products such as tofu "veggie" burgers and patties. Refer back to the section on protein for serving sizes and nutrition food labels.
  o When choosing beans for your selection of protein, make sure to check off one starch and one protein in you food journal.

- Try to use fats sparingly, also known as having in moderation.

  o Fats include all kinds of oils, butter, margarine, and many salad dressings. Remember that fat is concentrated in calories, so make sure you watch how much you are having. You really don't need to worry too much about adding it to your meals and snacks, especially when you cook with it or have foods higher in fats like nuts and avocados. Also, most animal products contain a certain amount of fat. Check nutrition food labels for serving sizes.

Conserving Calories

When planning your meals, try to conserve your calories. Cutting back on calories in easy places will help make a big impact on the amount of weight lost over time. In order for you to lose one pound, you have to have a calorie deficit of approximately 3500. For example, in order to lose half a pound per week, you would have to cut about 250 calories per day of what your body needs to function. To lose one pound per week you would have to cut about 500 calories each day. You can cause the calorie deficit by cutting calories from your meal plan or burning it off through exercise. Ideally you want to do both so that your body does not adjust to a very low amount of total calories and to build up your metabolism through exercising. Each calorie counts. By cutting back a little each day, you can easily lose at least one pound each week, but don't shoot for two, remember your metabolism. This is best done by avoiding empty calories and consuming more nutrient-dense, low-calorie foods.

"What are empty calories?" you may be asking. These are the little calories that easily add up when we are not careful. They are considered empty because they contain few if any nutrients. So basically they only contribute calories and little if anything else. Nutrient-dense foods pack a hefty amount of nutrients while being low in calories.

Tips:

- Eliminate regular soda, drinks, lemonades, and iced teas made with regular sugar. Basically, avoid any beverages with calories except for skim or 1% milk. Most beverages like regular sodas have at least 100-150 calories per serving. Stick with water or seltzer, and save the calories for something tastier and more filling. When you do have a craving for something besides water, try a diet soda or other calorie-free beverage instead, in moderation.

- Avoid drinking juice and stick with eating the fruit instead. OK, there are some juices out there that are not considered empty calories. Many are rich in nutrients; however, they still have anywhere from 100-150 per eight ounces. If you absolutely must have a glass of juice, then have it. Make sure that you measure it out, and look for a product that is all natural, preferably with no added sugar, and does not contain high fructose corn syrup. (I could go into detail as to why this bad for you; however, it would be another book.) Oh, and because a calorie is a calorie is a calorie, you have to count each half glass as one carbohydrate because each half glass (four ounces, not eight ounces) has about the same amount of calories and carbohydrates as, say, a piece of bread. Want to make those four ounces feel like more? Then mix your juice with seltzer to make it go longer.

- Avoid sports drinks and energy bars if possible unless there is nothing else available to eat or if you work out for more than an hour each day. These calories can and do add up. Instead, when you know you will be working out, bring a healthy snack and a bottle of water to have with you for the workout.

- Replace the sugar in your coffee and tea with a nonnutritive sweetener that is calorie free. Every teaspoon of regular sugar you have contains 16 calories. That was teaspoon I said, not tablespoon, which has 46 calories each. This doesn't sound like much, but let's say you have two to three cups of coffee or tea each day (and hopefully some of that is decaffeinated). If you were to put one tablespoon in each one, that is 138 additional calories per day from pure, refined sugar. Even if you use honey, it is the same thing, at least calorie wise. Remember a calorie, is a calorie is a calorie. When ordering your favorite flavored latte or cappuccino, ask for sugar-free syrup flavoring instead of regular, which can save you 20 calories per serving (and believe me, there is more than one serving in there).

- Try to avoid adding cream to your coffee or tea. Use skim milk instead. Each tablespoon of cream has about 50 calories and 5 grams of fat. You can easily pour in two to three (or more) servings if you are not paying attention. In comparison, a whole glass of skim milk has 80 calories and no fat. When you order a latte or cappuccino, ask for skim or soy milk instead of whole milk.

- When having pancakes, waffles, or French toast, go for regular old maple syrup and measure out no more than one tablespoon. For every tablespoon you use, check off one starch on your food journal. You could also use sugar-free syrup instead and save about 60-150 calories per serving depending on the syrup you use.

- Avoid empty foods like candies, chocolates, cookies, cakes, pastries, and pies; save them for special occasions only. Also, be careful of fat-free deserts that are also low in nutrients and can be high in calories. Fat-free desserts are fine in moderation, if you can stick to the appropriate serving size. The calories also add up. If you find that you are eating double the amount of cookies just because they are fat free, then you really haven't cut any calories. If fact, you may even be eating more than if you just stuck to the serving size of the regular version.

- Enjoy alcoholic drinks in moderation. Stick with serving sizes when you do have them, and try to avoid mixed drinks that can have added calories via

juices and mixes used. If using hard liquor, mix with seltzer or diet soda instead. One serving of alcohol is the equivalent of:
- 12 ounces of beer
- 5 ounces of wine
- 1.5 ounces of liquor

Boredom

When changing your eating habits, it is also very easy to get in a rut. Often, you find foods that seem to work and continue to eat them each and every day. This can lead to boredom with your meal plan and may lead you to eat foods you have been trying to avoid or have less of. Stop eating the exact same thing day after day. Instead, include a variety of foods in your meal plan.

For example:

- Try dishes you have never tried before. There are many cultures out there with unique and delicious dishes. By following the basics, you can enjoy these foods without going overboard on your calories.

- Liven up dishes by using ingredients that you normally wouldn't use. Try various herbs and spices to marinate protein-rich foods without adding salt, fat, or excess calories. Marinate in freshly squeezed lemon, limes, or oranges to tenderize foods without the excess salt.

- Vary your fruits and vegetables by sticking to the ones that are in season. This way you optimize your nutrient intake, constantly try new foods, and obtain the freshest ingredients.

- Invest in subscribing to cooking magazines that are geared for healthier living to help you try new dishes. Try to choose at least one (or more) new recipe to try each week.

- Purchase cookbooks geared at healthier living. However, buyer beware! Make sure that you check out the qualifications of the writer of the book. Anything by a registered dietitian (with the credentials RD after the name) is a good thing to look for. When the writer is an RD, you can assume that they went through extensive training to earn those credentials. Many books not written by an RD will have at least consulted an RD. Investigate!

- Try new recipes from various cooking shows on television. Use the basics you learned from Part I to adjust recipes that are calorie laden to make adjustments.

Mini Meals

As stated earlier, consume five or six meals per day instead of three large meals. Try to make each meal a mini meal, or have three main meals and two or three lighter meals (or snacks) per day. I don't expect you to count every calorie; however, start reading labels so that you know how many calories are in many of the foods you consume. Each main meal should consist of roughly of 300-400 calories (or less), and snacks should be about 200-300 (or less), depending on your body's daily calorie needs. Again, this doesn't mean that you are expected to count calories strictly. Just make sure that you are not eating 500-600 or more calories each meal, which can add up to 3000-3600 calories if you consume six meals per day.

You may be wondering how you are going to fit five to six meals in each day, and how such small meals are going to fill you up. The trick is how far apart you eat these meals and snacks. Ideally, you want to have your meals or snacks about every three to four hours apart. Wait no more than four to five hours in between meals at the maximum. Eating this often throughout the day will help prevent you from overeating, because you will rarely be ravenously hungry. By the time you start to get hungry again, it will be time for another meal or snack. This method of eating will take some getting used to; however, after a few weeks, your hunger and cravings will adjust, and the small meals will satisfy you. Give it a good two to three weeks for adjustment. For some of you it may take longer to adjust, and some of you will adjust in less than a week. Each person's period of adjustment will vary.

Along with having your meals every three to four hours, it is important to note that you need to eat something, also known as breakfast, within one to two hours after waking up in the morning. Your mother was right; breakfast is the most important meal of the day! Breakfast is the meal that will set you up for the rest of the day. After a long (or in some cases short) night of sleeping, your body needs some fuel to get it going. Your body's metabolism does slow down during the night; however, the body still needs to be recharged with food (not just sleep) to prepare for the day ahead. Your cell phone doesn't work without a charged battery, and neither does your body. It also prevents you from feeling like you are starving when lunchtime arrives, thus preventing unnecessary binges.

Make sure to have breakfast within one to two hours maximum after you wake up in the morning. Try to choose something rich in complex carbohydrates and some protein to keep you going until the next meal or snack. If you find that you are not hungry for breakfast, then you may be eating too much at night. Check out the chapter on breakfast options for some ideas.

Taking Your Time

Did you ever walk in the door of your home and begin eating without even taking notice of what you put in your mouth? Did you ever start eating without realizing that you were even eating? Often, we sit down for a meal (if we even sit) and eat the entire meal in a matter of minutes without even tasting the food. This pattern of eating can lead to weight gain if done on a consistent basis.

For many of us, this is how we eat most of our meals. For example, let's say you scarf down your food in ten minutes, have a second helping in the next five5 minutes, and then the third in ten minutes after that, you will have eaten three times what you would have normally have eaten if you just took a full twenty minutes to eat the first plateful. Often, we help ourselves to a second helping or even a third without a second glance. It can take up to twenty minutes for the brain to get the message that the body is full. By taking the full time to eat your meals, you will give the body a chance to send the right messages to the brain so that you don't overeat.

Eating in a rush can also have other consequences besides overeating. I'm talking about heartburn, folks. Most of you have experienced heartburn at some point in your life, especially if you suffer from GERD (gastroesophageal reflux disease). Here is the lowdown on heartburn. Between your mouth and your stomach is a tube called the esophagus.

Between that tube and your stomach is a flap that works hard at keeping things in the stomach and out of the tube where they don't belong. When there is too much pressure in the stomach, that flap has to work pretty hard at keeping everything in.

Let me put it in perspective for you: Thanksgiving is here, and you are off to dinner at your relative's house. You have large (and multiple) portions, much more than you usually would. On top of that, the foods that you consume probably have more fat than you eat day to day. Don't forget the cocktail with the appetizers and the wine with dinner. So now this food is sitting like a brick in your stomach, but here comes dessert and coffee. After the meal is complete, you lay back on the couch with a mint in your mouth and begin to enjoy the third or fourth football game of the day, burping away.

Talk about pressure in the stomach. Not only have you had too much to eat (causing pressure in the stomach) and heavy food that will hang out longer, but you added alcohol, caffeine, and mints to the mix. These are all foods that can lower the flap's defenses. To top it all off you laid down and let gravity make this flap work even harder. Now the burping will help make some room, but as you burp the flap loosens—and say hello to acid, a funny taste in your mouth, and fun chest pain.

With that said, the longer you take to eat, the less your risk of heartburn from overeating and the less belching ("gas"), which is oh, so charming, you will suffer. Also, the longer you take to eat, the faster you will get full, and thus the less food you will eat. Hopefully, you will be gradually adjusting well to the five or six mini meal plan, so this extreme hunger will soon be a thing of the past and won't hit you all of a sudden. Until you get to that point, there are a few things to remember so that if hunger hits, you don't go overboard:

Ways to slow things down:

- Drink a glass of water before you sit down for your meal and make sure that you are well hydrated in between meals and snacks. If you are having five to six meals and/or snacks each day, the five or six glasses of water you will be having before each meal will help you meet your fluid requirements. Also, sip on some water in between each bite.

- Eat your dinner at the dinner table instead of in bed (unless it is a special occasion) or on the couch. No room in the kitchen for a table or no dining room in your house? Try to invest in some tray tables to have your meals on. Make sure to shut off the television, put away any reading material, and stay off the phone so that you can concentrate. Pay attention to the food that is before you. Savor each and every bite of the meal. Oh, and turn off the computer, and don't answer any phone calls, texts, or e-mails!

- Digestion begins in the mouth. Make sure to chew each and every bite of food completely.

- I can't say this enough, so I will say it again. Try to allow yourself at least twenty minutes for each meal and ten minutes for each snack. After you finish what is on your plate, get up and walk around, use the bathroom, clean up the dishes, or take the garbage out. You probably won't need another helping. If after the twenty minutes you are still hungry, then by all means, have a little more.

Listen to Your Body

IMPORTANT NOTE:

If you have been diagnosed with depression or an eating disorder, or suspect that you suffer from depression or an eating disorder, the advice presented does not replace the advice of your health care provider.

Have you ever eaten something and wondered why you ate it? Did you ever sit down in front of the television with a bag of chips to find that moments later you had devoured most of the bag? Have you ever received a phone call in the middle of dinner to find that your plate was empty by the time the call ended? Were you really even hungry?

These days, not only do we eat too quickly, but more often we eat when we really aren't even that hungry. There are various reasons why people eat other than hunger. Often, we eat for the wildest reasons; unfortunately most of those reasons are not from hunger. In my many years as a registered dietitian, I have heard many of the excuses for eating, but often it just boils down to stress.

Stress often appears from life's little happenings. Any situation that is out of your control can lead to mental strain. It is this tension and anxiety that can cause many of us to eat just to cope with the out-of-control circumstances that creep up. Our nerves get the better of us and derail our good intentions to eat healthily.

I have yet to have a client say, "I can't believe I ate a whole bag of baby carrots!" Unfortunately, when we become "emotional eaters," we don't reach for the carrots and celery sticks. What is an "emotional eater"? This is a person who eats from various emotions such as sadness, anger, solitude, anxiety, disappointment, or depression. In a nutshell, from stress. If you are not careful, stress can spoil all of the positive changes you have worked so hard to make.

If you find that you are an "emotional eater," first you have to tap into the reasons and situations that cause you to become the "emotional eater." It is important to note that women are not the only "emotional eaters" out there. There are plenty of men out there who are just as guilty of letting stress lead the way to the kitchen pantry.

Besides "emotional eaters" there are those who eat tucked away, hidden from family and friends. Mainly, these "closet eaters" fear what people may think if they see what and how much they are eating. I have had many acquaintances in my career tell me that they eat nothing all day except for a bowl of cereal for breakfast, a salad for lunch, and some soup for dinner, and they just can't fathom why they are struggling with their weight. What they are not telling me about is all the extras that they didn't count, like the pastry with the coffee before the cereal, the candy bar from the vending machine before lunch, the cheese and ladlefuls of dressing on the salad, the regular soda on the side, and dessert and coffee after the soup. I think you get the point. "Closet" eating is just as dangerous as "emotional" eating.

The first thing to break the habit of "emotional" and "closet" eating is to write down everything that you are eating, no matter what it is. Everything must be written down, even the bite of food that you had from your friend's dish at lunch. Even if you had a bite and didn't like it, it must be written down. If you had it while standing up, then write it down (so you might as well sit). Remember, this food journal is for your eyes only. It is your tool to help you eat healthily. If you eat something and don't write it down, it is only you that suffers.

At the end of the day, or the next morning, take a few minutes to review everything that you ate. If there is anything that you had that you normally wouldn't have, or if it was a particularly stressful day, then write down what was going on. Start to spot any trends that begin to occur. You may have to look back a few days to spot trends. For example, if your mother notoriously calls in the middle of dinner, causing you to polish off a second and third helping of the meal, then don't answer the phone. Call her later, when you have left the kitchen, and tell her you were eating dinner. After a few nights, she will get the hint not to call at dinnertime, and if she doesn't, well, that is what voicemail is for.

Quiet! Listen for a minute. Your body is talking to you. Are you listening? Before you start eating something, especially if you just ate in the last hour, ask yourself, "Am I really hungry?" Or are you eating for some other reason? Are you stressed out, upset, or nervous? After writing down your feelings in your food journal, you should start to spot areas of trouble and be able to stop and take a moment to tune into the signals your body is sending you. If you are truly hungry, then by all means, eat something. Please remember to take your time and enjoy the meal.

If you are like many humans nowadays, your life is bombarded with an exceptionally high level of stress.

We live in a fast-paced society, where things are done faster than they ever were before. Mobile phones ensure that anyone can find you at a moment's notice. We carry laptops to coffee shops so that we can get work done while enjoying a cup of coffee. We now have mobile phones that also contain our date books in one place so we can make sure to book up our day. There is a price to this convenience. All of these gadgets allow us to multitask, which can mean multi-pressure. Stress is a part of our lives; however, there are things that you can do to unwind:

- Search for activities that promote relaxation.

- At the end of the day, treat yourself to a bubble bath. Make sure to turn off the telephone or mobile phone so you don't hear it. Put on some soft music; instrumentals work best because lyrics can make the mind wander. Set aside at least twenty to thirty minutes in the tub to completely unwind. Treat yourself to pleasant, scented bath soaps or gels and candles to make the experience even more enjoyable.

- Turn off the ringer to the house telephone or mobile phone when sitting down to dinner. The worst thing you can do for your meal plan is to talk on the telephone while you're eating, especially if it is bad news on the line or someone you really don't want to talk to. Just turn them off and deal with them after dinner when you are already full.

- Turn off the ringer to the house phone and your mobile when going to bed. Most people know not to call after a certain hour at night or too early the next morning. Despite this, there is always that one friend that decides to call you at eleven p.m. because they happen to be awake. Do yourself and your friendship a favor, and turn off the ringers. If you feel you need to keep them on for emergencies, then set them to low or vibrate. If they can't get you on the first try, then they will try again, and it should eventually wake you up.

- Set aside time to exercise most days of the week. Yes, we have been over this earlier in the book; however, I feel that it is so important that it needs to be repeated. This should be your time to zone out from the everyday and concentrate on your workout only. I have been to the gym many a time and seen people on their hands-free devices on their mobile phones on conference calls and booking appointments. While I applaud these folks for fitting physical fitness into their busy days, if possible try not to do work when you work out.

- Try relaxing activities and exercise routines like yoga and meditation. The best thing I did for my marriage was to start yoga when I entered graduate school. I decided at the age of twenty-eight to get my master's degree full time so I could complete it before I was thirty (because I wanted to start having children by then). I did this while still working five part-time jobs (talk about stressful multitasking). By the end of the day, my body was in a ball of knots. Someone recommended I try yoga to unwind. I started with one day a week in a yoga studio and worked up to two days each week in the studio and one to three days a week at home with a DVD. Needless to say, I got through it.

- Treat yourself to a monthly or bimonthly massage. This sounds expensive but is worth the cost if it allows you to unwind and get some sleep. Just make sure you go to someone who is licensed especially if you suffer from any physical ailments. If unsure, check with your healthcare provider. Often they have contacts they can send you to.

- Have your nails done. Yes, even the men out there can get your nails done. Treat yourself each week or every other week to feel pampered.

Not only will treating yourself to relaxing activities promote stress release, but if the occasional treat motivates you to stay on track, then all the more reason to do it. And besides, you deserve it. Treat yourself to something that you normally don't treat yourself to or haven't done in a long time. If you noticed, none of the treats are food related. The key is making sure you don't treat by rewarding with food.

Planning Your Meals and Eating Out

It can be difficult to eat healthily, especially when the bulk of your day is spent away from home. You many even consume four to five of your daily meals at work or some other location outside your home. This does not mean that it is impossible to eat healthy. It just means you have to plan a little more.

Every night before you head on up to bed, make sure that you have all of your meals prepared and packed away in the refrigerator for the next day. Try to do this at night and not the next morning when you are trying to get out the door. This also applies to those of you that work from home or are stay at home parents. By preparing your meals for the next day the night before, you will save time; however, that is not the only benefit. It can also save you a lot of money. Bringing your food to work or even out to the mall with you will save you money. On the road, restaurants located at rest stops are usually higher in price than the establishments located in the towns along the way. Many restaurants now offer healthier choices on the menu but often come at a hefty price. At times, the healthier choice can cost double or more than the other calorie- and fat-laden choices.

To get started, invest in:

- Small food storage containers with lids (preferably microwave and freezer safe). Look for 1-2 cup size containers to help with portion control.

- A small cooler or insulated lunch bag. This will help keep perishable foods fresh until you get to your destination or throughout the day if there isn't a

137

refrigerator available. Make sure to use ice packs to keep the packages cold.

- Reusable water bottle that holds 2-4 cups depending on your preference.

- Small sandwich bags or sandwich container (freezer safe).

Each time you cook, make more than you anticipate serving for the meal. If there are four of you in the family, then make enough for six or eight (depending on how many lunch bags you have to pack for the next day). If you dine alone, make an extra two to three servings of the dish you are preparing. Pack one serving for your lunch and place any extra servings in freezer-safe containers or bags. You can even do this before you sit down to eat to prevent yourself from eating any extras after you finish what is on your plate.

You can use the extras in the freezer for days when you didn't cook the night before, did not make enough food, or for any time you are home and don't feel like cooking. Consider them your homemade frozen dinners. This will help you cut back on salt, calories, and fat because you are controlling what you put into your frozen meals. Also, think of the money you'll save. If you are really short on time, then pick one day of the week and make a few dishes at once. Pack each dish in one or two serving-size containers (you can use one for dinner and one for lunch the next day. This way you are set for the week.

I'm not saying you can't use the already prepared frozen meals on the market, just do so in moderation (not every day). When shopping for them, check for sales and coupons (they always go on sale) and check for the healthier options. The product should be a single serving size container and contain three hundred to four hundred calories or less per serving and less than ten to fifteen grams of total fat per serving; and if possible, try to find a product with greater than four grams of fiber. If you can't, then you can add a fiber-rich food to the meal like an extra vegetable or half a cup of beans.

Besides lunch, pack at least one or two snacks for the day. If you know that you will be out for breakfast as well, then pack breakfast, too. This way you have the day covered in case you are running late or sitting in traffic. Now, it is best to sit down, relax, and have a meal, but sometimes that is not possible. Something to eat, even if it is in your car, is better than nothing at all. Just make sure that it is safe to do so.

Restaurant Dining

Even though you are trying to eat healthily, you don't have to only eat home-cooked meals. There are going to be times when you don't feel like cooking and want someone else to cook for you, and that is just fine. As long as the majority of your meals are prepared at home, you can occasionally partake in take out, or even fast food.

You can eat out and still eat healthily. Eating out can be a pleasurable experience, so go out and enjoy. This doesn't mean that you throw all you have learned out the window. Don't forget what you've learned up until now. The basics apply to foods cooked at home or in a restaurant. You can use all you have learned to enjoy a healthy meal without going off your meal plan.

If you have a day's notice, try to cut back during the day so that you can let loose a little for the meal that you are going to have out whether it is at a restaurant, fast food establishment, or party. This does not mean that you should starve the whole day. If you know that you are going out for lunch, try to plan for a light breakfast like cereal and milk, and snack on vegetables in between. That night have a lighter dinner like soup and a light salad. If the meal out will be breakfast or dinner, then adjust the other meals accordingly.

If you know where you are going to eat, have in mind what you are going to eat when you get there. Have a game plan. Many restaurants have their menu their Web sites, or they are more than happy to fax a menu to you. Many even provide you with nutrition information. If not, don't fret. You can use the basics that you have learned to get by.

A few tips for dining out:

- Before you even arrive at the restaurant, have a healthy snack at home to fill you up a bit before you get there. Getting to a restaurant starving is like grocery shopping when you are hungry. You will start eating whatever is placed down in front of you, like breadsticks or chips, and will likely order the first thing you see. Have something light like a light yogurt with a serving of peanuts mixed in.

- Stick with water or seltzer with lemon. Avoid sodas and mixed drinks that can rack up the calories and still leave you hungry. Stick with a diet soda that is calorie free. If you really want that regular soda, ask for lots of ice and only have one regular soda; then switch to water, seltzer, or diet soda. If you want to have something with alcohol, then stick with either a glass of wine, a twelve-ounce beer, or 1½ ounces of liquor mixed with seltzer or diet soda.

- Start your meal with a broth-based soup and steer away from cream-based soups. Cream soups are just that, cream based. Remember, one tablespoon of cream has fifty calories and five grams of fat. Usually, a small, one-cup bowl has more than one tablespoon of cream per serving.

- If soup is not your thing or you're just not in the mood for it, then start off with a vegetable-only salad. Ask your server to leave off any extras like croutons, bacon bits, or cheese. Vegetables only. If you are unsure what comes in the salad, then ask. Order your dressing on the side, and ask for a low-fat or nonfat dressing if available. If your dressing of choice is not available, then ask for olive oil and vinegar on the side.

- If you have the option of having a half-size portion, then order the half-size portion. If the option is small, medium, or large, then order the small. If you went for a cheeseburger, why are you getting the super duper sized economy meal? Remember to listen to your body. If the burger is what you came for, then that is what you should get.

- Look for menu items that allow you to choose your own sides, and then order only the vegetables (preferably non-starchy if having dessert). Order plain, steamed vegetables instead of sautéed or fried options.

- If you order anything that comes with sauces or extra condiments like butter or sour cream, ask for them on the side. Often you can get away with using only half of what is brought out to you, if you even use it.

- Ask for whole-grain options when available, like whole-grain bread or brown rice. When faced with a choice of potato, order it baked instead of fried or mashed.

- If the restaurant does not offer half-size portions, try to eat only half of what is brought out to you. Unless by chance you find an establishment these days that serves appropriate serving sizes, have your server provide you with a take-out container, and put half of the meal in the container before you even start to eat, unless you have the willpower to make sure that you only eat half.

- Want to order dessert? Try to stick with fresh fruit options or sorbets instead of sherbet or ice cream. If the cheesecake or crème brûlée is calling your name, then go for it. Remember, you can have it in moderation. If possible, share it with a friend, especially if it is a large portion.

Eat What You Crave

As I have said previously, this is not a "diet" book. There are no "forbidden foods." There are no "good" or "bad" foods here, just poor choices. You can pretty much fit almost anything into your daily meal plan. If your daily meal plan is filled with regular soda all day, sugar-laden cereals, and fast food, then you are making poor nutrition choices. However, if you eat a high amount of fruits, vegetables, whole grains, and low-fat animal products with an occasional slice of apple pie, then you are making predominately healthy choices. The most important thing to remember is to have foods that are loaded with calories or are nutritionally empty in moderation. This means once in a while, not once in a while every day, or with every meal.

Make a list of all the foods you usually overeat or splurge on, and put these on one side of a table or chart. Next, in the second column write some alternatives to these foods that would allow you to enjoy them on a more regular basis without wrecking your good intentions (see table 10 for an example).

Table 10: Food Substitutes

Food Item	Alternatives
Chocolate bar	Buy the mini versions or a full-size bar and cut into bite-size pieces. When you get home, place them in the freezer. Take out only one piece each day to enjoy. This way you know you are going to have it and can look forward to the treat. Eventually, you will probably forget it is there.
Ice Cream	Try having a frozen fruit bar or low-fat or nonfat ice cream or yogurt.
Cheese fries	Buy frozen french fries and bake them instead of frying. Better yet, peel, slice, and bake your own. Stick to the suggested serving size. Measure out one ounce of reduced-fat cheese, melt over the fries, and enjoy.
Milkshakes	Make your own with eight ounces skim milk and half a cup of low-fat or nonfat yogurt or ice cream and blend.
Nachos	• Buy baked tortilla chips and count or weigh one serving. Look for whole-grain items that can have up to four grams of fiber per serving. • Drizzle two tablespoons salsa and one ounce sharp cheddar cheese over one-fourth a cup black beans or vegetarian refried beans. • Heat in the microwave one to two minutes or until cheese has melted.
Potato Chips	Baked potato chips. Make sure to measure out one serving on the scale (one ounce of chips). Pretzels (one serving) Light or natural popcorn (one serving)

Whatever you do, don't completely avoid having the foods you love and crave. This is a way of life, not a temporary "diet." This is how you will be eating for the rest of your life. When you take all of the foods that you normally love and crave from your meal plan, you leave your body wanting them more and more. It isn't worth it to tell yourself that you will never have another piece of chocolate cake just for the sake of fitting into smaller jeans. It's not worth it if it means that next week you're going to want cake so badly that you will eat half the cake instead of just allowing yourself a slice that day.

Don't follow the all-or-nothing approach. If you eat eggs sausage, and pancakes for breakfast, then have a lighter lunch and dinner. Make sure you stick with portion sizes, or have less than a full portion size so that you can have it more often. Always remember, no food is forbidden.

Oh No! A Plateau!

Now you have been following a healthy meal plan for months and losing weight pretty consistently, when suddenly the weight loss stops. What do you do when you hit a weight plateau and the scale hasn't changed in weeks? How do you know that you have hit a plateau?

A plateau in the world of weight loss is when the weight loss stops and the inches are not budging even though you are still following your healthy changes and new exercise habits perfectly. If the inches are dropping but the scale isn't budging, you haven't hit a plateau; you're probably adding muscle to your body and getting rid of fat. That does count. But if the numbers on the scale and the measuring tape are staying the same, there are a couple of things you can try to get the numbers to go down again:

- You could continue what you are currently doing without changing a thing and wait to see if the plateau ends on its own. Usually, the plateau can lower your motivation and send you back to habits you thought you would never have again. So please keep reading.

- Your other option, which I recommend, is taking a look at your food journal and checking to see if there are any further changes you can make.

  o Are you having "treats" too often?
  o Are you slacking when it comes to exercise?
  o Have you been doing the same type of exercise without a variation? Do you need to change your exercise routine? Work out at a higher pace or intensity, for a longer amount of time,

and/or try some new form of exercise. Often, trying something completely new can get your metabolism moving.

o Are your portions too large or even too small? Too small?! Remember, when you are not eating enough calories, your body adjusts by getting used to a smaller amount and thus may cause you to plateau and even gain weight in some instances. You don't want your body to start running in starvation mode.

o Is this possibly the weight that you are meant to be at? You may not be losing any more weight because there isn't any more to lose. Just keep going with your healthy eating plan and exercise routine to keep off the weight you have lost and prevent you from regaining it. Head over to your health-care provider if you are not sure.

If you've tried everything above and are advised that you still need to lose more weight, then I highly suggest that you consider visiting with a registered dietitian to determine what may be off. Your local dietitian can spot things you may be missing in your food journal. Make sure to bring it with you so a better assessment can be made. Your dietitian's job is to help you, don't be worried that you may be laughed at or ridiculed for food you are eating. As a registered dietitian myself, I wish more people would come in with at least three to seven days' worth of logs in a food journal. This would give me a better idea of the foods a person likes and dislikes, and it would help me better assist you. Trust me, doing this will help you get more for your money.

If after visiting your health-care provider and registered dietitian, it has been concluded that you are at a healthy weight and eating plan, then keep up the good work! There is no reason to stop. Keep on following the basics, implementing what you have learned, trying new foods, relaxing, and treating yourself (not with food).

PART III:
Sample Menus:
Main Meals and Snacks

Day 1

Breakfast
- ½ cup bran flakes
- ½ cup skim milk
- 1 ¼ cups whole strawberries, sliced

- 6 ounces of hot tea or coffee
- ½ cup skim milk
- 1-2 packets of nonnutritive sweetener (optional)

Lunch
- 2 slices of whole-wheat bread
- 3-4 ounces of prepared tuna salad (see recipe idea that follows)
- romaine lettuce
- 1-2 ounces of sliced tomatoes
- 1 cup of cubed papaya

- Place romaine lettuce slices on one of the slices of wheat bread.
- Next, layer slices of tomatoes.
- Place tuna on bed of vegetables, and top with the other slice of wheat bread.
- Serve with cubed papaya.

Prepared Tuna Fish Salad
- *3 6-ounce cans of chunk light tuna packed in water*
- *¼ cup of chopped shallots*
- *1 cup sliced and chopped celery*
- *3 tablespoons freshly squeezed lemon juice*
- *½ cup light or low-fat mayonnaise*
- *1-2 teaspoons of Cajun seasoning*

- *Open all three cans of tuna and drain water from in each can.*

- *Add remaining ingredients and mix completely.*
- *Refrigerate for 1-2 hours until completely chilled.*
- *Makes approximately 6-8 servings.*

Dinner
- 3-4 ounces of roasted chicken, preferable the breast, skin removed (see recipe idea that follows)
- ⅔ cup of cooked rice (white or brown, whichever you prefer)
- ½ cup of black beans served over the rice (see recipe idea that follows)
- 1 cup tomato and onion salad (see recipe idea that follows)

Basic Roasted Chicken
- *5-6 pound roasting chicken*
- *Juice of 1 lemon or lime*
- *Juice of 1 orange*
- *1 can of low-sodium, fat-free chicken broth*
- *1 tablespoon of olive oil*
- *1 tablespoon of honey*
- *5-6 cloves of garlic, crushed and chopped*
- *Salt and pepper to taste*

- *Preheat the oven at 350ºF.*
- *Place the roasting chicken in a baking dish.*
- *Combine the remaining ingredients in a bowl and add to the chicken, making sure to marinate inside the chicken cavity as well.*
- *Bake until the until a meat thermometer reads 180°F, basting frequently (about 1½ to 2½ hours).*

Easy Black Beans
- *2 tablespoons olive oil*
- *1 medium onion, chopped*
- *4-5 cloves of garlic, smashed and chopped*
- *1 green pepper, chopped*
- *1 1/2 teaspoons dried oregano*

- *1 teaspoon cumin*
- *2-3 bay leaves*
- *2 cans of black bean soup (preferably something low in fat and salt if you can find it)*

- Heat up the oil in a 5-quart saucepan over medium heat.
- When the oil is hot, sauté the onions, garlic, and pepper until the onions are translucent.
- Add the oregano, cumin, bay leaves, and beans. Heat until cooked through and then serve.

Tomato and Onion Salad
- *2 beefsteak tomatoes, sliced thin*
- *1 medium onion, sliced into thin rounds*
- *1 tablespoon olive oil*
- *Salt and pepper to taste (or a low sodium seasoning)*

- Arrange tomato and onion slices on a serving dish. Drizzle with olive oil, and season to taste.

Day 2

Breakfast
- Spread 1 tablespoon of peanut butter on 1 slice of whole-wheat toast and top with half a large banana or 1 small banana.
- Enjoy with a mug of Café con Leche (see recipe idea that follows).

Café con Leche (Coffee with Milk)
- *2-3 ounces of prepared espresso*
- *1 cup of skim milk (or soy milk), steamed*
- *1-2 packets of nonnutritive sweetener*
- *1 serving of light nondairy whipped topping*
- *Ground cinnamon*

- *Place nonnutritive sweetener at the bottom of a medium-size coffee mug.*
- *Pour in espresso followed by the steamed milk.*
- *Top with whipped topping.*
- *Sprinkle with cinnamon and serve.*

Lunch
- 1 cup of the leftover black beans from the night before
- 1 ounce of cheese melted over the beans
- 1-2 ounces of sliced avocados served on top drizzled with jarred salsa (2 tablespoons)

Dinner
- Buffalo Chicken Salad (see recipe idea that follows).
- ½ cup of mango slices

Buffalo Chicken Salad

- *Remainder of chicken from the night before (remove all bones and skin and chop)*
- *2 tablespoons buffalo wing sauce (cayenne pepper sauce) for every cup of chopped chicken you have remaining.*
- *¼ cup of low-sodium, fat-free chicken broth for every cup of chopped chicken you have remaining.*
- *2 tablespoons of low-fat or nonfat bleu cheese dressing.*

- *Heat up the remaining chicken in a nonstick pan sprayed with nonstick cooking spray, and add the chicken broth.*
- *Stir in buffalo wing sauce. Cook until completely heated all the way through.*
- *While the chicken is heating up, prepare a salad consisting of vegetables only (try spinach leaves for a change, grape tomatoes, sliced red onions, chopped celery, and cucumbers).*
- *Top with 3-4 ounces of the cooked buffalo chicken and 2 tablespoons of low-fat or nonfat bleu cheese dressing.*

Day 3

Breakfast
- Southwest Breakfast Quesadilla (see recipe idea that follows)
- 1 orange

Southwest Breakfast Quesadilla
- *1 whole-grain tortilla (1-ounce size)*
- *½ cup prepared black bean salsa (or ½ cup of remaining black beans prepared from Day 1)*
- *1 ounce grated pepper jack cheese (or 1 ounce of your favorite cheese)*

- *Heat a nonstick sauté pan sprayed with nonstick cooking spray.*
- *While pan is heating, cut the tortilla in half.*
- *Place the salsa on one half and top with grated cheese.*
- *Top with the other half of the tortilla.*
- *Grill on each side until the cheese is melted and the tortilla is toasted.*

Lunch
- Buffalo Chicken Sandwich (prepared with the ingredients listed below)
    - 3-4 ounces of the leftover buffalo chicken salad that you made last night
    - 2 slices of whole-wheat bread or a whole-grain English muffin
    - 1 leaf of romaine lettuce
    - 1-2 ounces of sliced tomatoes
    - 1 tablespoon low-fat or nonfat bleu cheese dressing
- Celery sticks (about 3 ounces)
- Apple slices (1 small, 4-ounce apple)

Dinner
- 3-4 ounces of beef tenderloin (see recipe idea that follows)
- ⅓ cup of rice (white or brown) mixed with ½ cup of leftover black beans (if beans are done, either make more or have an extra ⅓ of rice)
- 1 cup steamed broccoli
- 4 ounces of orange juice over ice, topped off with lime-flavored seltzer and crushed mint leaves

Beef tenderloin
- *2 pounds of beef tenderloin (cut into 5- or 6-ounce pieces)*
- *½ head of garlic gloves, crushed and chopped*
- *½ cup of flat leaf parsley*
- *¼ cup of olive oil*
- *Juice of 1 large orange*
- *Juice of 2 limes*
- *Salt and pepper to taste*

- *Place all of the ingredients in a storage bag (gallon size) and allow to marinate for at least 4 hours.*
- *Grill on a grill pan or in a BBQ.*
- *Serve immediately.*

Day 4

Breakfast
- ½ cup of old-fashioned, quick-cooking oatmeal
- ½ cup skim or soy milk (or water)
- 1-2 tablespoons of peanut butter
- 1 small banana (or ½ a large banana), sliced into small pieces

- Place oatmeal, milk (or water), and peanut butter in a small bowl.
- Heat in the microwave for 1 minute.
- Slice bananas over oatmeal and serve.

Lunch
- Mini whole-grain bagel
- 1 veggie burger (heated in the microwave according to package directions)
- 2 tablespoons jarred salsa
- 1 ounce sliced avocado
- 3 ounce of baby carrots
- ¾ cup fresh pineapple chunks

- Prepare veggie burger and place on mini whole-grain bagel.
- Top with avocado and salsa.
- Serve with baby carrots and pineapple chunks on the side.

Dinner
- 1 cup cooked pasta (any shape you like), prepared according to manufacturer's directions.
- ½ cup of prepared marinara sauce (jarred is just fine)
- ¼ cup nonfat ricotta cheese mixed with
- ¼ cup nonfat cottage cheese

- Vegetable salad
- 1-2 tablespoons of low-fat or nonfat Italian dressing
- 1 kiwi, sliced

- Combine all of the ingredients above and heat in microwave.
- Serve with a vegetable salad with 1-2 tablespoons of low-fat or nonfat Italian dressing and sliced kiwi.

Day 5

<u>Breakfast</u>

<u>Morning Smoothie</u>
- 1 cup of skim milk or soy milk
- ½ cup plain, nonfat yogurt (can be substituted with plain soy yogurt)
- ½ cup fresh or frozen berries
- 1-2 packets of nonnutritive, calorie-free sweetener (optional)

Blend all ingredients in a blender or food processor, pack into a travel mug, and enjoy while getting dressed in the morning.

<u>Lunch</u>
Since dinner is out tonight, lunch is 1 can low-fat, low-sodium soup (variety of choice), sprinkled with 1 ounce cheese and paired with 1 cup cubed cantaloupe and honeydew mixture.

<u>Dinner (out at a local steakhouse)</u>
Many steakhouses offer a salad to start with, so if this is the case order the garden salad instead of the Caesar salad—and make sure to ask the server what is in the salad. Make sure that you insist on vegetables only. Ask for any low-fat or nonfat dressings available and ask for them on the side. If low-fat or nonfat is not available, then ask for olive oil and vinegar on the side.

For drinks, try to stick with water or seltzer. If you want a beer or a glass of wine, then go for it, but try to stick to one or the other and just one.

For the main meal order, look for the leanest cut of meat available. Search for words like round, sirloin, and tenderloin and order the smallest cut available (usually six ounces is the smallest available). If you are able to order your own sides, try to order two non-starchy vegetables if possible. If the baked potato is calling your name, then go for it and ask for the condiments (sour cream, butter, bacon bits, and shredded cheese) on the side.

Want dessert? Stick with fresh fruit or a sorbet if available; if not, then go for what you really want and try to split it with a friend.

Day 6

<u>Breakfast</u>

Morning Wrap: This dish can be prepared the night before and reheated in a panini grill, toaster oven, or heated in the microwave while you are getting ready for work. Have it for breakfast, lunch, dinner, or a snack.

<u>Morning Wrap</u>

- *1 whole-grain Tortilla (1-ounce size)*
- *1 ounce Swiss cheese (or 1 ounce of your favorite cheese)*
- *2 egg whites (or ¼ cup egg white substitute), pan cooked in Pam cooking spray*
- *1 portion of lite sausage or vegetarian sausage (prepared according to microwave directions (sliced in half, length wise)*
- *¼ cup chopped tomatoes or prepared salsa*

- *Place tortilla flat on a plate.*
- *Place Swiss cheese, egg whites, lite or vegetarian sausage, and chopped tomatoes on one end of the tortilla and fold into a wrap making sure to fold in sides to prevent filling from falling out.*
- *If prepared the night before, reheat in a toaster oven or panini grill.*

<u>Lunch</u>

- 2 slices of whole-wheat bread (toasted)
- 1 ounce reduced-fat vegetable cream cheese (or suggested serving size)
- 2-3 ounces smoked salmon (make sure to check the date on the package you purchase and try to use within 1-2 days of purchase)
- Red onions (sliced in rounds)

- Cucumbers (sliced thin)
- Tomatoes (sliced thin)
- ½ a large grapefruit

- Spread ½ of the cream cheese on each slice of toast.
- Layer smoked salmon, red onions, cucumbers, and tomatoes.
- Enjoy with grapefruit sections on the side.

Dinner
- 3-4 ounces modified meatloaf (see recipe idea that follows)
- 1 cup prepared mashed potatoes (replace butter with vegetable or chicken broth)
- ½-1 cup sautéed chopped asparagus (1 inch pieces), see recipe idea that follows
- 1 fresh peach

Modified Meatloaf
- *1 cup white beans*
- *½ cup low-fat, low-sodium chicken, beef, or vegetable broth*
- *2 cups onions, roughly chopped*
- *3-4 garlic cloves*
- *½ chopped parsley*
- *1 teaspoon dried oregano*
- *1½ pounds 90-95% lean ground beef (you can also substitute lean ground chicken, lean ground turkey, lean ground pork, or any combination of the four meats)*
- *1 tablespoon olive oil*
- *Bread crumbs from 1-2 slices of whole-wheat bread (finely ground in a dry blender or food processor)*
- *Salt (optional) and pepper to taste*
- *1 whole egg*

Glaze (combine all and whisk together)
- *¼ cup ketchup*
- *1 tablespoon maple syrup*
- *1 tablespoon hoisin or low-sodium soy sauce*
- *¼ teaspoon allspice (Asian variety)*
- *Pepper to taste*

- *Preheat the over to 350°F degrees if you plan on baking the meatloaf immediately.*
- *In a blender or food processor, puree the beans, broth, onions, garlic, parsley, and oregano.*
- *Combine the mixture with the grounds meats, olive oil, and egg until well mixed. Add breadcrumbs. How wet the loaf is determines how many slices of bread you need to use. You don't want it too dry or too wet. If you are able to make a ball out of the mixture without it falling apart, then you have added enough.*
- *Place in a bread pan that has been sprayed with nonstick cooking spray. Place in the oven and bake for 45 minutes to an hour until a meat thermometer reads 160°F. Approximately 20 minutes into cooking, spread the glaze on top for the remainder of the cooking time.*

Sautéed Chopped Asparagus
- *1 bunch asparagus chopped into 1-inch pieces, blanched*
- *1 tablespoon olive oil*
- *1 tablespoon light soy sauce*

- *Heat olive oil in a nonstick sauté pan.*
- *When heated, add asparagus pieces and sauté for 2-3 minutes.*
- *Add soy sauce and cook for another 2-3 minutes and serve.*

Day 7

Breakfast
- 1 frozen whole-grain waffle
- 1 tablespoon peanut butter
- 1 tablespoon pure maple syrup
- ½ cup berries (or any fresh fruit in season)

- Heat waffle according to package directions.
- Spread peanut butter over heated waffle.
- Place berries over peanut butter and drizzle with maple syrup.
  - *To save on calories and/or sugar, use sugar-free syrup or sugar-free fruit spread.*

Lunch
- Leftover Meatloaf Sandwich
  - ½ of whole-grain pita
  - 2 ounces leftover meatloaf
  - 1 slice Swiss cheese
  - 1 leaf romaine lettuce
  - 1-2 ounces sliced tomatoes
- 1 cup mixed blackberries and raspberries

Dinner
- 4 ounces BBQ breast (see recipe idea that follows)
- 1 medium corn on the cob
- 1 cup steamed broccoli
- 1¼ cups cubed watermelon

BBQ Chicken
- *1 pound chicken breast (3-4 ounces each, no bones)*
- *¼ cup prepared BBQ sauce*
- *Juice of 1 lime*
- *1 tablespoon olive oil*

- *Combine all of the ingredients in a large food storage bag (gallon size) and allow to marinate for at least 4 hours.*
- *Heat a grill pan and spray with nonstick cooking spray, and grill until chicken reaches a temperature of 180ºF degrees.*

Snack Ideas

Black Bean Salsa
- 1 can of black beans, rinsed and drained
- 1 can corn, rinsed and drained
- 1 pint of grape or cherry tomatoes
- ½ cup chopped red onions
- Juice of 2 limes
- 1 tablespoon olive oil (optional)

- Combine all ingredients in a bowl
- Refrigerate for 1-2 hours before serving.
- Serving size is ½ cup.

Enjoy with:
1 ounce whole-grain tortilla chips, 3 ounces celery sticks, 1 ounce whole-grain bagel chips, or as a condiment on burgers or burritos.

Power Yogurt
- 1 cup fresh fruit
- 8 ounces plain (nonfat) or light yogurt (whichever flavor you fancy)
- 1 ounce of chopped nuts (whichever you like the most)
- Granola bar

I don't know about you, but plain yogurt never filled me up. I smash up a plain old granola bar and have it with 1 cup of plain or light yogurt and fresh fruit.

Peanut Butter and Fruit
Spread 1 tablespoon of peanut butter on a small apple or banana.

Cheese and Crackers

Measure out 1 ounce of any crackers (preferably a whole-grain cracker that has at least 2 grams of fiber). Look for products that have large serving sizes like 10-15 crackers. They may be smaller, but then you can make mini sandwiches with them with 1 ounce of your favorite sliced cheese.

Cereal Standby

When you are on the go, busy at work, or with the kids, cereal is a healthy quick fix for a meal or a snack. However, I know it rarely fills me up for more than 2 hours. Enjoy 1 cup (or the suggested serving size on the label) with ½ cup (or 1 cup) of skim or soy milk. Look for cereals with at least 3-5 (or more) grams of fiber per serving.

Garlic Bread

- 1 large whole-wheat baguette, sliced into ¼- to ½-ounce pieces
- 3 tablespoons olive oil
- 1½ tablespoons white wine
- 4 garlic cloves, crushed and chopped
- 3-4 tablespoons chopped fresh Italian parsley (or 1-2 teaspoons dried parsley
- 1 teaspoon dried oregano
- Grated Parmesan cheese

- Preheat the over to 325ºF degrees.
- Combine olive oil, vinegar, garlic, parsley, and oregano in a small bowl.
- With a kitchen brush, brush each piece of bread with oil mixture and sprinkle Parmesan cheese over bread (about ½ teaspoon each piece).
- Heat in toaster oven until cheese melts (about 10-13 minutes).
- Enjoy 2-4 pieces of them as a snack or with a meal.

Veggie Plate
- 3 ounces sliced cucumbers
- 3 ounces baby carrots
- 3 ounces grape tomatoes
- 1-2 tablespoons low-fat or nonfat dressing of choice
- 1 ounce cheese of choice, sliced

- Drizzle the dressing over prepared vegetables and enjoy with cheese.

Gelatin Surprise:
- 2 cups frozen berries
- 1 package sugar-free gelatin mix (choose the flavor that matches the fruit will be using)

- Place ½ cup of frozen berries in 4 serving dishes.
- Prepare sugar-free gelatin as directed in package directions, and divide between the 4 dishes.

References:

1. Gerberding, J.L., Marks, J.S. Mokdad, A.H., & Stroup, D.F. (2004). Actual Causes of Death in the United States, 2000. *JAMA,* 291 (10), 1238-1245.

2. Centers for Disease Control and Prevention. (2009, August 19). *Overweight and Obesity: Health Consequences.* Retrieved January 11, 2010, from http://www.cdc.gov/obesity/causes/health.html

3. *Cabbage Soup Diet Information.* Retrieved January 11, 2010, from http://www.cabbage-soup-diet.com

4. United States Department of Agriculture. (2009, April 6). *Inside the Pyramid: How much Physical Activity is Needed?* Retrieved January 12, 2010, from http://www.mypyramid.gov/pyramid/physical_activity_amount.html

5. U.S. Department of Health and Human Services: U.S. Food and Drug Administration. (2009, June 18). *How to Understand and Use the Nutrition Facts Label.* Retrieved December 15, 2009, from http://www.fda.gov/Food/LabelingNutrition/ConsumerInformation/UCM078889.htm#

6. Centers for Disease Control. (n.d.). *Eat a Variety of Fruits and Vegetables Every Day: What Counts as a Cup.* Retrieved December 23, 2009, from http://www.fruitsandveggiesmatter.gov/what/examples.html

7. Local Harvest. (n.d.). *Food Coops.* Retrieved December 8, 2009, from http://www.localharvest.org/food-coops/

8. American Dietetic Association & American Diabetes Association. (2008). *Choose Your Foods: Exchange Lists for Diabetes.* (pp. 13-16).

9. Whole Grains Council. (n.d.). *Whole Grains 101.* Retrieved January 8, 2010, from http://www.wholegrainscouncil.org/whole-grains-101

10. Whole Grains Council. (n.d). *Health Studies on Whole Grains.* Retrieved January 11, 2010, from http://www.wholegrainscouncil.org/whole-grains-101/health-studies-on-whole-grains

11. United States Department of Agriculture: National Agricultural Library. (2009, October 23). *Dietary Reference Intakes: Macronutrients.* Retrieved December 8, 2009, from http://fnic.nal.usda.gov/nal_display/index.php?info_center=4&tax_level=3&tax_subject=256&topic_id=1342&level3_id=5140

12. Whole Grains Council. (n.d). *Whole Grain Stamp.* Retrieved January 11, 2010, from http://wholegrainscouncil.org/whole-grain-stamp

13. U.S. Department of Health and Human Services: U.S. Food and Drug Administration. (2009, October 22). *Food and Drug Administration Modernization Act of 1997.* Retrieved December 18, 2009, from http://www.fda.gov/RegulatoryInformation/Legislation/FederalFoodDrugandCosmeticActFDCAct/SignificantAmendmentstotheFDCAct/FDAMA/FullTextofFDAMAlaw/default.htm

14. Department of Health and Human Services (HHS) & Department of Agriculture. (2005). *Chapter 5: Food Groups to Encourage.* Retrieved January 11, 2010,

from
http://www.health.gov/dietaryguidelines/dga2005/do
cument/html/chapter5.htm

15.   American Dietetic Association & American
        Diabetes Association. (2008). *Choose Your Foods:*
        Exchange Lists for Diabetes. (pp. 7-12).

16.   U.S. Department of Health and Human Services:
        U.S. Food and Drug Administration. (2009, October
        29). *Fresh and Frozen Seafood: Selecting and Serving*
        it Safely. Retrieved January 12, 2010, from
        http://www.fda.gov/Food/ResourcesForYou/Consume
        rs/ucm077331.htm

17.   The American Egg Board. (n.d.). *Learn More*
        About Eggs: Nutrient Breakdown. Retrieved January
        12, 2010, from
        http://www.aeb.org/LearnMore/NutrientBreakdown.ht
        m

18.   Morning Star Farms. (n.d.). *Dietary Needs.*
        Retrieved January 10. 2010, from
        http://www.morningstarfarms.com/dietary_choices.a
        spx?healthy=43

19.   National Dairy Council. (2005). *Dietary*
        Guidelines & Food Guidance System. Retrieved
        December 28, 2009, from
        http://www.nationaldairycouncil.org/EducationMateria
        ls/DietaryGuidance/Pages/Dairysrole.aspx

20.   American Dietetic Association & American
        Diabetes Association. (2008). *Choose Your Foods:*
        Exchange Lists for Diabetes. (pp. 17-19, 28-35).

21.   Breakstone's. (n.d.) *Product Info: Breakstone's Cottage Cheese Small Curd 4% Milkfat*. Retrieved January 12, 2010, from http://brands.kraftfoods.com/Breakstones/main.aspx?s=product&m=product/product_display&Site=1&Product=2100012283

22.   Breakstone's. (n.d.) *Product Info: Breakstone's Cottage Cheese Small Curd 2% Milkfat*. Retrieved January 12, 2010, from http://brands.kraftfoods.com/Breakstones/main.aspx?s=product&m=product/product_display&Site=1&Product=2100030047

23.   Department of Health and Human Services (HHS) & Department of Agriculture. (2005). *Key Recommendations for the General Population*. Retrieved January 11, 2010, from http://www.health.gov/dietaryguidelines/dga2005/recommendations.htm

24.   Mayo Foundation for Medical Education and Research. (2009, January 31). Retrieved November 13, 2009, from http://www.mayoclinic.com/health/fat/NU00262